Study Guide for

Textbook of

Reproductive Medicine

Second Edition

This study guide includes continuing medical education material, an educational activity sponsored by:

SOUTHWESTERN
THE UNIVERSITY OF TEXAS
SOUTHWESTERN MEDICAL CENTER
AT DALLAS

ACCME Accreditation

The University of Texas Southwestern Medical Center at Dallas is accredited by the Accreditation Council for Continuing Medical Education to sponsor continuing medical education for physicians.

AMA/PRA Credit Designation

The University of Texas Southwestern Medical Center at Dallas designates this educational activity for a maximum of 30 hours in Category I credit towards the AMA Physician's Recognition Award. Each physician should claim only those hours of credit that he or she actually spent in the educational activity.

This CME activity was planned and produced in accordance with the ACCME Essentials.
Date of original release: April 1998; Term of approval: 3 years

See page 215 for additional CME instructions.

The University of Texas Southwestern Medical Center at Dallas Office of Continuing Education

DISCLOSURE OF SIGNIFICANT RELATIONSHIPS WITH RELEVANT COMMERCIAL COMPANIES/ORGANIZATIONS

Study Guide for Textbook of Reproductive Medicine, 2nd Edition April 1998

According to the University of Texas Southwestern "Disclosure Policy," faculty involved in continuing medical education activities are required to complete a "Conflict of Interest Disclosure" to disclose any real or apparent conflict(s) of interest related directly or indirectly to the program. This information is acknowledged solely for the information of the participant.

The faculty listed below have disclosed a financial interest or other relationship with a commercial concern related directly or indirectly to the activity (names of companies are listed after each presenter's name). Those presenters not listed have disclosed no financial interest or relationship.

UT Southwestern does not view the existence of these interests or relationships as implying bias or decreasing the value of the presentation.

This educational activity has been planned to be well-balanced and objective in discussion of comparative treatment regimens. Information and opinions offered by the authors represent their viewpoints. Conclusions drawn by the reader should be derived from careful consideration of all available scientific information. Products may be discussed in treatment of indications outside current approved labeling.

Faculty

Bruce R. Carr, MD	Author of *Study Guide for Textbook of Reproductive Medicine, 2nd Edition,* 1998
Richard E. Blackwell, PhD, MD	Author of *Study Guide for Textbook of Reproductive Medicine, 2nd Edition,* 1998

Study Guide for

Textbook of

Reproductive Medicine

Second Edition

Bruce R. Carr, MD
Paul C. MacDonald Professor of Obstetrics and Gynecology
Director, Division of Reproductive Endocrinology
Department of Obstetrics and Gynecology
University of Texas Southwestern Medical Center at Dallas
Dallas, Texas

Richard E. Blackwell, PhD, MD
Professor of Obstetrics and Gynecology
Department of Obstetrics and Gynecology
University of Alabama at Birmingham
Birmingham, Alabama

Instructions for obtaining CME credit appear on page 215.

APPLETON & LANGE
Stamford, Connecticut

Copyright © 1998 by Appleton & Lange
A Simon & Schuster Company

98 99 00 01 02 / 10 9 8 7 6 5 4 3 2 1

Prentice Hall International (UK) Limited, *London*
Prentice Hall of Australia Pty. Limited, *Sydney*
Prentice Hall Canada, Inc., *Toronto*
Prentice Hall Hispanoamericana, S.A., *Mexico*
Prentice Hall of India Private Limited, *New Delhi*
Prentice Hall of Japan, Inc., *Tokyo*
Simon & Schuster Asia Pte. Ltd., *Singapore*
Editora Prentice Hall do Brasil Ltda., *Rio de Janeiro*
Prentice Hall, *Upper Saddle River, New Jersey*

Acquisitions Editor: Jane Licht
Production Editor: Sondra Greenfield
Production Service: Rainbow Graphics, LLC
Developmental Editor: Beth P. Broadhurst

ISBN 0-8385-8894-8

PRINTED IN THE UNITED STATES OF AMERICA

Contents

Preface

Prior to the preparation of the second edition of the *Textbook of Reproductive Medicine*, we decided to prepare a study guide. The study guide includes questions for each chapter of the text, pertinent case reports as well as an additional 100 questions for continuing medical education credits (30 hours).

We hope this Study Guide adds significantly to the education of our readers.

Bruce R. Carr, MD
Richard E. Blackwell, PhD, MD

Acknowledgments

We would like to thank our administrative staff for the preparation of this Study Guide and Case Reports. We wish to express our thanks to Darlene Farmer (Dr. Carr's administrative assistant) and Murrill Lynch (Dr. Blackwell's administrative associate).

I

DEVELOPMENTAL CHANGES IN REPRODUCTIVE MEDICINE

Chapter 1

FERTILIZATION, EMBRYOGENESIS, AND IMPLANTATION

1–1. Following mitotic proliferation, human fetal oocytes enter into meiosis and arrest at the following stage:

    a. metaphase II
    b. prophase II
    c. diplotene I
    d. none of the above

1–2. Resumption of meiotic maturation is controlled by

    a. increase in cyclic adenosine monophosphate (cAMP) and an increase in luteinizing hormone (LH peak)
    b. decrease in cAMP and a decrease in LH
    c. increase in LH and contact between granulosa cells and the oocyte
    d. decrease in cAMP and a loss of contact between granulosa cells and the oocyte

1–3. Which of the following has the most intimate or closest contact with the oolemma of the oocyte?

    a. granulosa cells
    b. thecal cells
    c. zona pellucida
    d. luteal cells

1–4. Spermatogenesis differs from oogenesis in that

    a. the spermatogonium undergoes mitosis and meiosis
    b. spermatogenesis is a continual, renewable process

    c. spermatogenesis is under follicle-stimulating hormone (FSH) and LH regulation
    d. the length of time to complete meiotic maturation is the same in spermatogenesis and oogenesis

1–5. Before the sperm can fertilize an oocyte it must do the following (second step):

    a. the spermatozoa display hyperactivation
    b. capacitation occurs
    c. an acrosome reaction occurs
    d. binding to the zona pellucida occurs

1–6. Which glycoprotein is involved in species-specific binding to the zona pellucida?

    a. ZP1
    b. ZP2
    c. ZP3
    d. ZP4

1–7. Formation of gap junctions between the cells occurs first at/in

    a. syngamy
    b. the morula stage
    c. blastomeres
    d. the inner cell mass

1–8. What types of distinct tissues do NOT form during implantation?

    a. cytotrophoblasts
    b. syncytiotrophoblasts
    c. inner cell mass
    d. neuroblasts

1–9. Which of the following is NOT a sperm surface receptor involved in fusion?

a. SP56
b. P95
c. α-mannoside
d. integrin

1–10. In which of the following human cell stages does the control of gene expression switch from maternal to zygote control?

a. 2 cell
b. 4 cell
c. 8 cell
d. morula

1–11. Which of the following appears to influence the formation of decidual endometrium?

a. activin
b. calcium
c. calmodulin
d. prostaglandin

1–12. The length of time that the human blastocyst resides in the uterine cavity is

a. 12 hours
b. 24 hours
c. 48 hours
d. 72 hours

1–13. Which of the following animals exhibits the largest delay in implantation of the blastocyst?

a. armadillo
b. sable
c. cat
d. dog

1–14. Which of the following does NOT regulate the accumulation of blastocoele fluid?

a. ovumorulen
b. prolactin
c. compaction of morula cells
d. appearance of tight junctions

1–15. What is the average number of days from initiation of spermatogenesis until sperm reach the caudal epididymis?

a. 20
b. 40

c. 70
d. 90

1–16. Which of the following is NOT a part of the cumulus–granulosa–oocyte complex?

a. acrosome reaction
b. zona pellucida
c. germinal vesicle
d. cortical granules

1–17. Which of the following is the correct sequence of sperm maturation and fertilization?

a. hyperactivation, capacitation, cortical reaction, penetration of zona
b. capacitation, hyperactivation, penetration of zona, cortical reaction
c. cortical reaction, hyperactivation, penetration of zona, capacitation
d. capacitation, penetration of zona, hyperactivation, cortical reaction

1–18. The surface of the zona pellucida

a. is solid
b. is fenestrated
c. is smooth
d. consists primarily of ZP1

1–19. The time required for sperm migration out of the seminal fluid following ejaculation is

a. 2 seconds
b. 10 seconds
c. 2 minutes
d. 10 minutes

1–20. Which structure lies between the plasma membrane and the zona pellucida of the ovum?

a. cortical layer
b. granulosa
c. cortical granule
d. perivitelline space

1–21. Restriction of the ability of a blastomere to form cell structures is called

a. expansion
b. determination
c. totipotency
d. accumulation

1–22. Which part of the blastocyst attaches to the endometrium?

    a. hypoblast
    b. inner cell mass
    c. syncytial trophoblast
    d. cytotrophoblast

1–23. The optimal time for replacement of donor oocytes is days

    a. 9 to 11
    b. 11 to 13
    c. 13 to 16
    d. 16 to 19

1–24. The length of time that the human blastocyst remains free in the uterine cavity before hatching is

    a. 24 hours
    b. 36 hours
    c. 72 hours
    d. 96 hours

1–25. Decidualization

    a. is progesterone dependent
    b. occurs at day 25 of the cycle
    c. occurs in endometrial stromal cells
    d. all of the above

1–26. Which of the following is NOT characteristic of oocyte metabolic activation?

    a. increased RNA
    b. calcium influx
    c. NA^+/H^+ exchange
    d. pH decrease

1–27. The mature sperm consists of all of the following EXCEPT

    a. haploid nucleus
    b. tail with axoneme $7 + 7 + 2$
    c. inner acrosome membrane
    d. acrosome

Chapter 2

THE ENDOCRINOLOGY OF PREGNANCY

CASE REPORT

A 22-year-old primigravida patient with phenotypic abetalipoproteinemia and genotypic homozygous hypobetalipoproteinemia presented in early gestation. The patient had been treated with vitamin E therapy since age 11, with a current diagnosis of abetalipoproteinemia. The only abnormality she had on physical examination was areflexia. She had been studied as a teenager and demonstrated to have an impaired adrenal response to a prolonged adrenocorticotropic hormone (ACTH) stimulation test. In addition, at approximately age 19, the patient underwent extensive hormonal evaluation throughout a menstrual cycle. During the menstrual cycle, the patient had frequent sampling of gonadotropins and serum progesterone. As seen in Figure 2–1, her luteinizing hormone (LH) and follicle-stimulating hormone (FSH) levels peaked at midcycle and were in the normal range. However, during the luteal phase, her progesterone levels were only slightly detectable.

Her total cholesterol was only 27 mg/dL and her low-density lipoprotein (LDL) cholesterol was <3 mg/dL (Table 2–1). It was believed that the patient exhibited a form of severe luteal-phase deficiency. Even though the patient had low progesterone levels, she continued to have regular cyclic menstrual periods.

At age 22, the patient conceived spontaneously and presented to her local physician at approximately 10 weeks' gestation. The patient was on prenatal vitamins as well as supplemental vitamin E and vitamin A. The initial examination revealed a pregnancy of appropriate size, which was confirmed by ultrasound. Growth of the uterus and fetus was normal by ultrasound at 31 and 38 weeks'

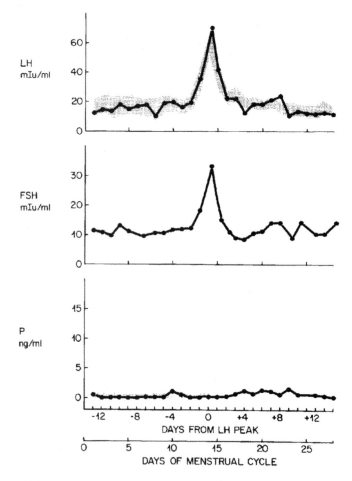

Figure 2–1. The levels of LH, FSH, and progesterone in a woman with hypobetalipoproteinemia during a menstrual cycle. Hatched area represents range in normal women. *(Reproduced, with permission, from the American Society of Reproductive Medicine. Carr BR, MacDonald PC, and Simpson ER. The role of lipoproteins in the regulation of progesterone secretion by the human corpus luteum. Fertil Steril. 38:303–311, 1982.)*

Table 2–1. Plasma Lipid Profile in a Woman Having Homozygous Hypobetalipoproteinemia

	Plasma Lipids (mg/dL)				
	Total-C	LDL-C	HDL-C	VLDL-C	TG
Nonpregnant					
Patient	27	<3	25	<3	7
Normal	175	105	50	20	90
Pregnant (term)					
Patient	35	<3	30	<3	4
Normal	238	139	55	54	150

gestation. At 31 weeks' gestation, urinary pregnanediol excretion revealed 16.5 mg per 24 hours, which is one third that of normal. The patient had an uncomplicated spontaneous labor at 42 weeks' gestation and delivered a 3370 g female infant with an Apgar score of 9/9 and no evidence of postmaturity. The umbilical cord and placenta were normal on gross examination and histologically. The infant was breast fed and given supplemental formula and had appropriate development.

Blood samples were obtained for estrogens and progesterone, as well as human placental lactogen and relaxin throughout pregnancy. The levels of progesterone and estradiol were markedly decreased compared to that of normal women (Fig 2–2). Levels

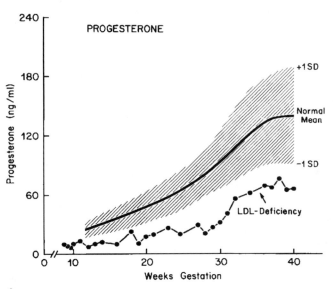

A

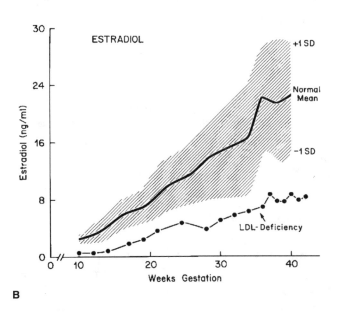

B

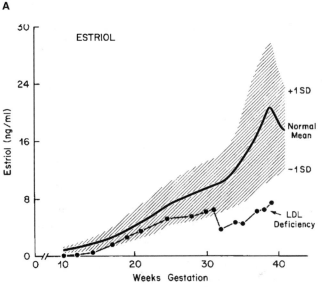

C

Figure 2–2. A–C. Serum levels of progesterone, estradiol, and estriol throughout pregnancy in a woman with homozygous hypobetalipoproteinemia. Values of patient are indicated by the solid circles. Values from normal women during gestation (hatched area) are mean ±1SD. *(Reproduced, with permission, from Parker RC Jr., Illingworth DF, Bissonnette J, and Carr BR. Endocrine changes during pregnancy in a patient with homozygous familial hypobetalipoproteinemia. N Engl J Med. 314:557–560, 1986.)*

Table 2–2. Umbilical Cord Plasma Lipoprotein Cholesterol (C) and Adrenal Steroids in a Newborn Having Heterozygous Hypobetalipoproteinemia

| | Lipoproteins (mg/dL) | | | | DS | F |
	Total-C	LDL-C	HDL-C	VLDL-C	ng/mL	μg/dL
Heterozygote	49	12	28	9	1500	20
Normal	60	33	23	4	2100	14

of estriol, on the other hand, were within normal range until late in pregnancy. Thereafter, the levels remained low until delivery. In contrast, maternal levels of human placental lactogen and relaxin were normal.

The patient's plasma lipids did not change from her nonpregnant values (see Table 2–1). In normal women, total cholesterol and LDL increase during pregnancy. Newborn cord plasma cholesterol levels, particularly LDL cholesterol levels, were subnormal as seen in Table 2–2. These findings were consistent with a predicted diagnosis of heterozygous hypobetalipoproteinemia in the infant. However, the umbilical cord plasma levels of cortisol and dehydroepiandrosterone sulfate (DHEAS) were within normal limits.

SUMMARY AND CONCLUSIONS

Results of this study confirmed the fact that plasma LDL cholesterol is an important source for cholesterol for steroidogenic tissues in humans. Previously, we have shown in vitro data that both the placenta and the corpus luteum require cholesterol in the form of LDL to reach optimal rates of steroid secretion of progesterone. In this particular patient, who demonstrated severe luteal-phase deficiency, no supplemental progesterone was given, but she demonstrated reduction in plasma progesterone, estradiol, and estriol. Since levels of human placental lactogen and relaxin (which are protein hormones secreted by the placenta) were normal, it is determined that the decline in steroid hormones was not due to reduced placental growth or function. The deficiency of progesterone, estradiol, and estriol can be correlated with the reduced source of LDL cholesterol substrate used for hormone synthesis. To us as investigators, it was remarkable that the patient ever became pregnant, let alone carried the pregnancy to term without any problem. The

role of progesterone, or at least the level required to maintain a normal pregnancy, is questioned by the clinical outcome of this study. In view of her low serum progesterone level during the luteal phase and during the first trimester of pregnancy, the role of luteal-phase defects as a cause of recurrent pregnancy abortion is also questioned. It is probably not the level of progesterone, but it may be the progesterone-to-estrogen ratio that may be critical in maintenance of normal pregnancy.

In addition, we demonstrated in the in vitro study that the placenta had an increased capacity of making cholesterol de novo, that is, an increased activity of hepatic hydroxymethylglutaryl coenzyme A (HMG CoA)-reductase compared to normal placenta (Fig 2–3). Under these circumstances, the placenta was able to make progesterone directly from two carbon units more efficiently than it would during normal pregnancy.

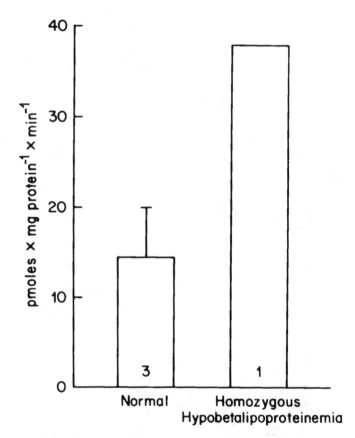

Figure 2–3. Level of HMG CoA-reductase activity in placental microsome preparations from the placenta of the subject and a normal pregnant subject.

BIBLIOGRAPHY

Carr BR, Sadler RK, Rochelle DB, Stalmach MA, MacDonald PC, Simpson ER. Plasma lipoprotein regulation of progesterone biosynthesis by human corpus luteum tissue in organ culture. *J Clin Endocrinol Metab.* 52:875, 1981

Illingworth DR, Alma NA, Sundberg EE, Hagemenas FC, Layman DL. Regulation of low-density lipoprotein receptors by plasma lipoproteins for patients with abetalipoproteinemia. *Proc Natl Acad Sci USA.* 80:3475, 1983

Illingworth DR, Connor WE, Buist NRM, Jhaveri BM, Lin DS, McMurry MP. Sterol balance in abetalipoproteinemia: studies in a patient with homozygous familial hypobetalipoproteinemia. *Metabolism.* 28:1152, 1979

Parker CR Jr., Illingworth DR, Bissonnette J, Carr BR. Endocrinology changes during pregnancy in a patient with homozygous familial hypobetalipoproteinemia. *N Engl J Med.* 314:557, 1986

Winkel CA, Snyder JM, MacDonald PC, Simpson ER. Regulation of cholesterol and progesterone synthesis in human placental cells in culture by serum lipoproteins. *Endocrinology.* 106:1054, 1980

QUESTIONS

2–1. During the first trimester of pregnancy, which of the following organs is the primary source of progesterone?

   a. corpus luteum
   b. ovarian follicle
   c. cytotrophoblast
   d. amnion

2–2. The placenta is deficient in which of the following enzymes?

   a. aromatase
   b. cholesterol side-chain cleavage
   c. 17α-hydroxylase
   d. 17β-hydroxysteroid dehydrogenase

2–3. Which of the following is the primary source of cholesterol utilized by the placenta for progesterone biosynthesis?

   a. LDL cholesterol
   b. high-density lipoprotein (HDL) cholesterol
   c. very low-density lipoprotein (VLDL) cholesterol
   d. total cholesterol

2–4. During human pregnancy, the levels of progesterone do not decline significantly in anencephalic pregnancies.

   a. true
   b. false

2–5. Which is the primary precursor for estriol formed by the human placenta?

   a. DHEAS
   b. androstenedione
   c. androstenedione sulfate
   d. testosterone

2–6. Estriol levels are low in all of the following pregnancies EXCEPT

   a. sulfatase deficiency
   b. anencephaly
   c. hydatidiform mole
   d. dexamethasone therapy

2–7. At which week of gestation does human chorionic gonadotropin (hCG) reach a peak?

   a. 3 weeks
   b. 10 weeks
   c. 20 weeks
   d. term

2–8. The α-subunits are similar in all of the following EXCEPT

   a. LH
   b. FSH
   c. thyroid-stimulating hormone (TSH)
   d. gonadotropin-releasing hormone (GnRH)

2–9. hCG has a structure similar to which of the following peptides?

   a. human placental lactogen (hPL)
   b. growth hormone (GH)
   c. prolactin (PRL)
   d. none of the above

2–10. PRL reaches a peak at midgestation in

   a. maternal serum
   b. fetal serum
   c. amniotic fluid
   d. umbilical vein blood

2–11. Which of the following hormones increases in maternal blood during pregnancy?

    a. cortisol
    b. angiotensin
    c. desoxycorticosterone (DOC)
    d. all the above

2–12. All of the following hormones reach a peak at midgestation in fetal blood and decline until term EXCEPT

    a. LH
    b. PRL
    c. GH
    d. FSH

2–13. Which of the following readily passes through the maternal to the fetal compartment?

    a. thyrotropin
    b. thyroxine
    c. propylthiouracil
    d. triiodothyronine

2–14. Which of the following hormones is secreted in the greatest amount by the fetal zone?

    a. DHEAS
    b. androstenedione
    c. cortisol
    d. corticosterone

2–15. One would anticipate the levels of LDL cholesterol and DHEAS in fetal blood in anencephalic pregnancy as follows:

    a. LDL low, DHEAS low
    b. LDL low, DHEAS high
    c. LDL high, DHEAS low
    d. LDL high, DHEAS high

2–16. The level of 17-hydroxyprogesterone in the second trimester of pregnancy is

    a. increased
    b. decreased
    c. increased 10-fold
    d. none of the above

2–17. Which of the following estrogens exhibits the highest level in maternal blood?

    a. estrone
    b. estetrol
    c. 17α-estradiol
    d. 17β-estradiol

2–18. All of the following are true regarding 16-OH DHEAS EXCEPT it

    a. is formed by fetal liver
    b. is converted to estrone
    c. decreases following betamethasone treatment of the mother
    d. is formed by the maternal liver

2–19. hPL levels are elevated in all of the following pregnancy conditions EXCEPT

    a. multiple gestation
    b. Rh disease
    c. diabetes
    d. preeclampsia

2–20. Amniotic fluid levels of prolactin at term compared to the second trimester are

    a. lower by one half
    b. higher by twofold
    c. the same
    d. extremely low

2–21. Which of the following is the first site of alphafetoprotein (AFP)?

    a. fetal nervous system
    b. fetal liver
    c. yolk sac
    d. none of the above

2–22. Which of the following is true regarding the neocortex, or definitive zone, of the fetal adrenal zone?

    a. It secretes primary DHEAS.
    b. It undergoes necrosis following delivery.
    c. It becomes the future adult cortex.
    d. It is the largest zone of the fetal adrenal gland.

2–23. The gene for the β-subunit for hCG is encoded on which chromosome?

    a. 6
    b. 8
    c. 14
    d. 19

2–24. During which trimester of gestation is the α-to-β ratio of hCG in maternal serum less than 1?

    a. first
    b. second
    c. third
    d. none of the above

2–25. Which chromosome contains the gene that encodes hPL?

    a. 6
    b. 8
    c. 17
    d. 19

2–26. Which of the following hormones is formed from progesterone by extra-adrenal enzymatic 21-hydroxylase activity?

    a. cortisol
    b. corticosterone
    c. DOC
    d. aldosterone

2–27. Which of the following hormones is low in maternal blood?

    a. ACTH
    b. corticotropin-releasing hormone (CRH)
    c. FSH
    d. relaxin

Chapter 3

PARTURITION

3–1. In the sheep model of parturition, the hormone of fetal origin that initiates labor is

    a. cortisol
    b. dehydroepiandrosterone (DHEA)
    c. androstenedione
    d. aldosterone

3–2. The enzyme that is activated in the sheep placenta that directs an increase in estrogen and a fall in progesterone levels is

    a. cholesterol side-chain cleavage
    b. aromatase
    c. 17α-hydroxylase
    d. 3β-hydroxysteroid dehydrogenase

3–3. Which of the following hormones has been shown to arrest labor in women?

    a. progesterone
    b. 17α-hydroxyprogesterone
    c. medroxyprogesterone acetate
    d. none of the above

3–4. Which of the following is thought to be the most likely rate-limiting step in prostaglandin formation?

    a. phospholipase activity
    b. prostacycline release
    c. arachidonic acid release
    d. prostaglandin E_2 (PGE_2) metabolism

3–5. Oxytocin is synthesized in the

    a. cerebral cortex
    b. intestine
    c. granulosa cell
    d. testis

3–6. Oxytocin receptors are present in high amounts in the

    a. myometrium
    b. cervix
    c. vagina
    d. brain

3–7. Oxytocin plays a major role in

    a. milk ejection
    b. onset of parturition
    c. cervical dilation
    d. cervical ripening

3–8. Endothelin is a class of peptides that cause

    a. vasodilation
    b. release of atrial natriuretic peptide
    c. vasoconstriction
    d. endometrial growth

3–9. Activation of smooth muscle myosin magnesium adenosine triphosphatase (MgATPase) activity requires

    a. phosphorylation of the light chain of myosin
    b. calmodulin formation
    c. phosphorylation of the heavy chain of myosin
    d. calcium binding

3–10. Which of the following assists in cervical ripening?

    a. collagenase
    b. interleukin-1 (IL-1)
    c. estrogen
    d. all of the above

3–11. The number of gap junctions in human myometrium before term is

    a. low
    b. high
    c. intermediate
    d. higher than during labor

3–12. Which of the following hormones regulates myometrial gap junctions?

    a. transforming growth factor-alpha (TGF-α), transforming growth factor-beta (TGF-β)
    b. estrogen, progesterone
    c. IL-1$_2$, IL-1β
    d. cortisone, corticosterone

3–13. Which of the following inhibits nitric oxide (NO) synthase?

    a. L-arginine
    b. L-nitro-arginine methyl ester (L-NAME)
    c. guanylate cyclase
    d. none of the above

3–14. NO is believed to play a role in parturition by which mechanism?

    a. vasodilator
    b. uterine relaxant
    c. uterine stimulant
    d. all of the above

3–15. The primary etiology to explain the onset of labor in women is

    a. the oxytocin theory
    b. progesterone withdrawal
    c. fetal signal
    d. unknown

3–16. Which of the following endogenous hormones is known to initiate parturition in humans?

    a. arginine vasopressin (AVP)
    b. progesterone
    c. oxytocin
    d. none of the above

3–17. Which of the following hormones is made de novo in sheep placenta but not human placenta?

    a. DHEA
    b. progesterone
    c. pregnenolone
    d. cholesterol

3–18. Which of the following is true in human pregnancy?

    a. ACTH infusion into fetus initiates labor.
    b. Progesterone levels fall prior to labor.
    c. The placenta lacks 17α-hydroxylase.
    d. all of the above

3–19. Which of the following enzymes when deleted (knocked out) in mice results in delayed parturition?

    a. aromatase
    b. 7α-hydroxylase
    c. 5α-reductase type 1
    d. 3β-reductase type 2

3–20. Which of the following is NOT true regarding prostaglandins?

    a. They act near tissue where they are produced.
    b. They act in tissue where they are produced.
    c. They often enter circulation as activated hormone.
    d. none of the above

3–21. Which of the following prostaglandins increases in concentration in amniotic fluid?

    a. PGE$_2$
    b. PGF$_{2α}$
    c. PGFM
    d. all of the above

3–22. Women who lack posterior pituitary function and oxytocin exhibit

    a. delayed onset of spontaneous labor
    b. failure to lactate and nurse
    c. infertility
    d. all of the above

3–23. Myosin is composed of

    a. two heavy-chain subunits
    b. one medium-chain subunit
    c. one light-chain subunit
    d. all of the above

3–24. In relaxed myometrial tissues

  a. cytoplasmic Ca^{2+} concentrations are elevated
  b. cytoplasmic Ca^{2+} concentrations are low
  c. Ca^{2+} is bound tightly to calmodulin
  d. myosin light-chain kinase is maximally activated

3–25. NO synthase inhibitors have which of the following effects in vivo?

  a. stimulate uterine contractility
  b. stimulate onset of parturition
  c. inhibit oxytocin release
  d. none of the above

3–26. During cervical ripening, all of the following occur EXCEPT

  a. qualitative changes in glycosaminoglycan
  b. increase in hyaluronic acid
  c. increase in collagenase
  d. decrease in water content in cervical tissues

3–27. Which of the following does NOT increase cyclic guanosine monophosphate (cGMP) levels in smooth muscle cells?

  a. oxytocin
  b. NO
  c. sodium nitroprusside
  d. nitroglycerin

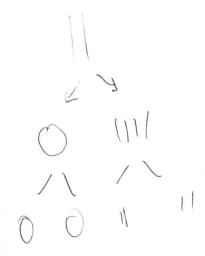

GENETICS IN REPRODUCTION

4-1. The secondary structure of deoxyribonucleic acid (DNA)

    a. provides a template for new DNA
    b. guards against damage
    c. includes coiling of 146 base pairs of DNA around histones
    d. allows compression of DNA

4-2. The cell cycle is composed in order of the following phases.

    a. G_0, S, G_1, G_2, M
    b. M, G_0, G_1, G_2, S
    c. G_0, G_1, G_2, S, M
    d. G_0, G_1, S, G_2, M

4-3. In mitosis, cytokinesis is characterized by

    a. dense chromosomes that align at the equatorial plate
    b. division of cell membranes into two daughter cells with 2n chromosomes
    c. division of cell membranes into two daughter cells with 4n chromosomes
    d. a resting phase

4-4. Meiosis includes which of the following stages in the correct order?

    a. leptotene, zygotene, pachytene, diplotene, diakinesis
    b. leptotene, zygotene, diplotene, pachytene, diakinesis
    c. metaphase, leptotene, diplotene, anaphase I, telophase I
    d. diplotene, diakinesis, anaphase I, telophase I, metaphase

4-5. At the end of meiosis II, which of the following exists?

    a. primary spermatocytes
    b. spermatids
    c. mature sperm
    d. secondary spermatocytes

4-6. Follicular atresia is first observed during fetal development at approximately week

    a. 12
    b. 16
    c. 20
    d. 24

4-7. Chromosome analysis can be performed on

    a. leukocytes
    b. fetal cells in amniotic fluid
    c. skin fibroblasts
    d. all of the above

4-8. The Y chromosome includes

    a. 20 million base pairs
    b. short arm (Yq)
    c. long arm (Yp)
    d. testis-determining factor (TDF)

4-9. Which of the following is believed to be primarily involved as the TDF?

    a. ZFY
    b. SRY
    c. H-Y antigen
    d. all of the above

4-10. Fertilization of gametes from a meiotic I error results in offspring with

    a. monosomy 25 percent, trisomy 50 percent, euploidy 25 percent
    b. monosomy 25 percent, trisomy 25 percent, euploidy 25 percent
    c. monosomy or trisomy
    d. all euploidy

4–11. Which of the following describes the background risk of neural tube defects in the United States?

   a. 4/1000
   b. 10/1000
   c. 1/1000
   d. 1/10,000

4–12. Amniocentesis can be performed at weeks

   a. 14 to 17
   b. 7 to 15
   c. 5 to 7
   d. a and b

4–13. Translation involves

   a. separation of double-stranded DNA into single strands
   b. complementary DNA (cDNA)
   c. formation of proteins
   d. DNA transcribed into ribonucleic acid (RNA) from 5′ to 3′ end

4–14. Which of the following is NOT a blotting technique?

   a. Eastern
   b. Western
   c. Northern
   d. Southern

4–15. Southern blotting uses which of the following?

   a. DNA
   b. RNA
   c. RNA probes
   d. protein

4–16. Disadvantages of in situ hybridization include which of the following?

   a. requires a known gene sequence
   b. requires a small sample
   c. uses a visual signal
   d. none of the above

4–17. Advantages of polymerase chain reaction (PCR) over Southern blotting include all of the following EXCEPT

   a. single copy
   b. results in 1 day

   c. used in cloning
   d. prevents contaminants with other DNA

4–18. Testicular feminization syndrome includes all of the following EXCEPT

   a. mapped to Xq 11–12
   b. due to a single gene defect
   c. involves the androgen receptor gene
   d. has variable phenotypes

4–19. Which of the following karyotypes is NOT characteristic of gonadal dysgenesis?

   a. 46,XX
   b. 46,XY
   c. 46,XXY
   d. 45,X

4–20. 45,X/46,XY individuals often have all of the following characteristics EXCEPT

   a. mixed gonadal dysgenesis
   b. born with sexual ambiguity
   c. gonads consist of ovotestes
   d. a gonad may consist of a unilateral streak

4–21. Which of the following is NOT a base component of DNA?

   a. uridine
   b. guanine
   c. thymine
   d. cytosine

4–22. Which of the following symbols is the appropriate nomenclature for the long arm of the chromosome?

   a. p
   b. i
   c. q
   d. l

4–23. In which of the following stages does the chromosome divide?

   a. interphase
   b. metaphase
   c. anaphase
   d. telophase

4–24. If parents are carriers for cystic fibrosis, what is the risk of offspring having the disease?

    a. 1:1
    b. 1:2
    c. 1:4
    d. 1:16

4–25. If a woman is a carrier for hemophilia A, what is the chance that her male child will have hemophilia A?

    a. 1:1
    b. 1:2
    c. 1:4
    d. 1:16

4–26. The staining technique to identify the chromosome that uses heating of chromosomes is

    a. H banding
    b. S banding
    c. R banding
    d. Q banding

4–27. Which of the following is NOT true regarding cystic fibrosis?

    a. most common mutation at DF_{508}
    b. carrier rate is 1 in 20 Caucasians
    c. X-linked disorder
    d. gene located on chromosome 7

4–28. Which of the following is true regarding Duchenne muscular dystrophy?

    a. dominant trait
    b. small gene
    c. incidence 1/5000 births
    d. linked to Xp21.2

4–29. Which of the following can be observed in the spectrum of androgen insensitivity due to disorders of androgen receptor?

    a. congenital sexual ambiguity
    b. female genitalia
    c. gynecomastia
    d. all of the above

4–30. Which of the following is observed in 45,X individuals?

    a. lymphedema
    b. horseshoe kidney
    c. cubitus valgus
    d. all of the above

4–31. Which of the following is indicated in a phenotypic classical Turner syndrome with 45,X?

    a. laparoscopy
    b. removal of gonad
    c. initiation of therapy with birth control pills
    d. none of the above

4–32. Which of the following is true regarding 45,X patients?

    a. origin of X chromosome is usually mother
    b. origin of X chromosome is usually father
    c. high frequency of undetected Y material
    d. eunuchoid features

Chapter 5

NORMAL AND ABNORMAL PUBERTY

CASE REPORT

A 2-year-old female patient presents with breast development, pubic hair, and menstrual bleeding. She had been born at term of an uncomplicated pregnancy. Growth and development was normal until 3 months prior to evaluation. Breast growth slowly increased over the past 3 months and pubic hair the past 2 months. One day prior to evaluation, menstrual bleeding was noted.

Physical examination revealed weight and height in the 95th percentile for her age. She demonstrated obvious breast development, Tanner stage II (Fig 5–1). Pelvic exam revealed Tanner stage I–II pubic hair development, and the vulva

was slight erythematous and moist. The remainder of the examination, including neurological, was normal. Initial laboratory results included a follicle-stimulating hormone (FSH) level of 4 mIU/ml, a luteinizing hormone (LH) level of 5 mIU/ml, and an estradiol level of 65 pg/ml, which was elevated for a prepubertal girl. A gonadotropin-releasing hormone (GnRH) stimulation test revealed a five- to tenfold increase in LH levels, which were indicative of a pubertal rise. Thyroid-stimulating hormone (TSH), prolactin (PRL), dehydroepiandrosterone sulfate (DHEAS), testosterone, and human chorionic gonadotropin (hCG) levels were normal. Bone age was slightly advanced (age 3).

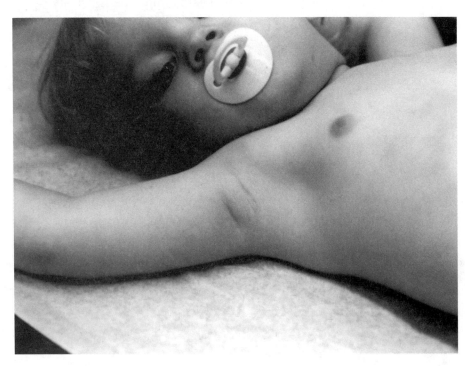

Figure 5–1. Photograph of a 2-year-old child demonstrating breast development. *(Courtesy of Dr. Karen D. Bradshaw, University of Texas Southwestern Medical Center at Dallas, Dallas, TX.)*

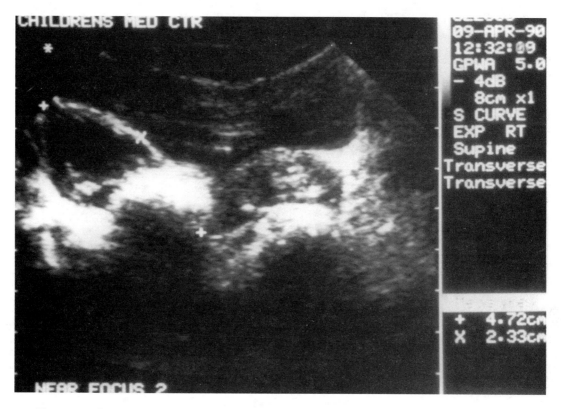

Figure 5–2. Pelvic sonogram revealing ovarian cyst. *(Courtesy of Dr. Karen D. Bradshaw, University of Texas Southwestern Medical Center at Dallas, Dallas, TX.)*

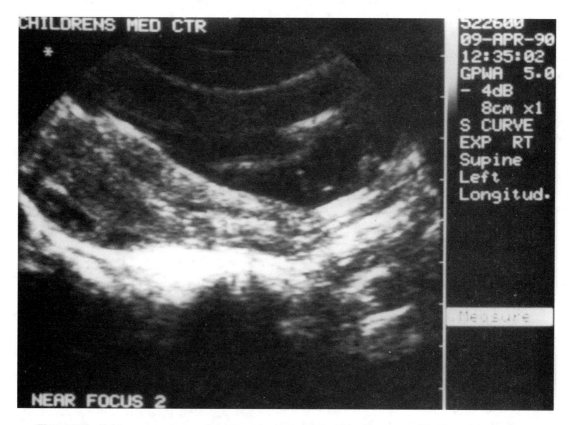

Figure 5–3. Pelvic sonogram revealing uterus-to-cervix relationship. *(Courtesy of Dr. Karen D. Bradshaw, University of Texas Southwestern Medical Center at Dallas, Dallas, TX.)*

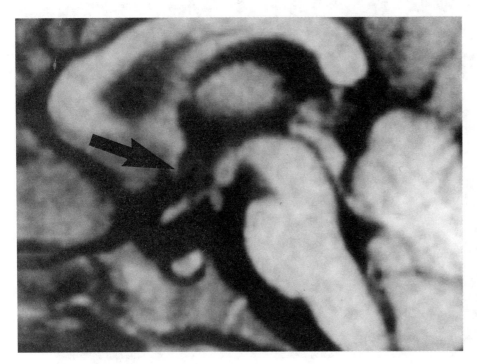

Figure 5–4. MRI of the head revealing small hamartoma above the tuber cinereum (see arrow). *(Courtesy of Dr. Karen D. Bradshaw, University of Texas Southwestern Medical Center at Dallas, Dallas, TX.)*

An abdominal sonogram revealed a 3 × 4-cm ovarian cyst and an enlarged uterus, which revealed an increased fundal-length-to-cervix ratio, compatible with pubertal development (Figs 5–2, 5–3).

A magnetic resonance image (MRI) was obtained, which revealed a 2-mm hypothalamic hamartoma in the region of the tuber cinereum (Fig 5–4). Due to the location and small size of the tumor, primary resection was not warranted. The child was started on a long-acting GnRH agonist every month, with rapid regression of breast growth and cessation of vaginal bleeding. Repeat ultrasound examination 2 months later revealed absence of ovarian cysts. The plan is to monitor the size and growth of the tumor by yearly head MRI and continue GnRH agonist therapy until age 10.

SUMMARY AND CONCLUSIONS

This child was diagnosed as a case of isosexual true sexual precocity. There are two types of true precocious puberty: (1) idiopathic or constitutional, in which no etiology can be detected; and (2) organic causes, including hamartomas, craniopharyngiomas, gliomas, and ependymomas. However, constitutional causes are more common, comprising up to 90 percent of cases of true precocious puberty.

Children with true precocious puberty develop pubertal changes in the progression of normal puberty, that is, breast development and growth, and pubic hair followed by ovulatory menses. However, the time of progression is often compressed, as in this case, over 3 months rather than 2 to 4 years. The LH response to GnRH is also exaggerated, as is observed in normal puberty, which supports a pre-awakening of the hypothalamic–pituitary axis. Evaluation includes measurement of sex steroids, hCG, TSH, and bone age; abdominal–pelvic ultrasound; and MRI of the head. Treatment of brain tumors is usually surgical except in very small hamartomas or those tumors that respond to suppressive therapy. In this case, treatment of pubertal signs and symptoms with GnRH agonists was successful. However, if the tumor continues to grow rapidly, then surgery may be required.

BIBLIOGRAPHY

Asherson RA, Jackson WPA, Lewis B. Abnormalities of development associated with hypothalamic calcification after tuberculosis meningitis. *Br Med J.* 2:839, 1965

Conn PM, Crowley WF. Gonadotropin-releasing hormone and its analogues. *N Engl J Med.* 324:93, 1991

Judge DM, Kulin HE, Page R, et al. Hypothalamic hamartoma: a source of luteinizing-hormone-releasing factor in precocious puberty. *N Engl J Med.* 296:7, 1977

Kaplan SL, Grumbach MM. Pathophysiology and treatment of precocious puberty. *J Clin Endocrinol Metab.* 71:785, 1990

Klech RP. Management of precocious puberty. *N Engl J Med.* 312:1057, 1985

Root AW, Shulman DI. Isosexual precocity: current concepts and recent advances. *Fertil Steril.* 45:749, 1986

Styne DM, Grumbach MM. Puberty in the male and female. Its physiology and disorders. In: Yen SSC, Jaffe RW, eds. *Reproductive Endocrinology. Physiology, Pathophysiology, and Clinical Management*, 2nd ed. Philadelphia, PA, W. B. Saunders, 1986: 313:350

QUESTIONS

5–1. Which of the following is in the correct chronological order of pubertal development in girls?

   a. growth spurt, breast bud, sexual hair, menarche
   b. breast bud, sexual hair, growth spurt, menarche
   c. breast bud, growth spurt, sexual hair, menarche
   d. sexual hair, breast bud, growth spurt, menarche

5–2. Which of the following best describes Tanner stage IV breast development?

   a. breast bud
   b. adult breast
   c. secondary mound
   d. nipple elevation

5–3. In order to obtain a bone age, which of the following is required?

   a. x-ray of epiphysis of knee
   b. Bayley–Pinneau tables
   c. Johnson–Bayley tables
   d. all of the above

5–4. The mean age of menarche in the United States is

   a. 11.8 years
   b. 12.3 years
   c. 12.8 years
   d. 13.3 years

5–5. During male puberty, gynecomastia may develop in

   a. 10 percent
   b. 20 percent
   c. 40 percent
   d. 60 percent

5–6. Adrenarche is best defined as

   a. onset of pubic hair
   b. onset of axillary hair
   c. increased DHEA/DHEAS levels
   d. increased cortisol levels

5–7. The average age of adrenarche in girls is

   a. 4 years
   b. 6 years
   c. 8 years
   d. 10 years

5–8. Which of the following is true if a 14-year-old girl fails to exhibit breast development?

   a. She will never menstruate.
   b. She likely has a microprolactinoma.
   c. An FSH level should be obtained.
   d. She is referred to a specialist.

5–9. The first laboratory test to be obtained in a 16-year-old girl with absence of sexual characteristics and pubertal development is

   a. β-hCG
   b. FSH
   c. PRL
   d. LH

5–10. If a 17-year-old patient fails to withdrawal bleed to a progestin challenge, which of the following is possible?

   a. pregnancy
   b. Asherman syndrome
   c. prolactinoma
   d. all of the above

5–11. Sexual precocity is defined in girls if signs of pubertal development occur before age

   a. 7 years
   b. 8 years
   c. 9 years
   d. 10 years

5–12. Which of the following is the most common cause of true (central) precocious puberty?

  a. hamartomas
  b. hypothyroidism
  c. McCune–Albright syndrome
  d. idiopathic

5–13. McCune–Albright syndrome is NOT associated with

  a. G_s abnormality
  b. absence of the catalytic unit of G proteins
  c. café au lait spots
  d. Cushing syndrome

5–14. A 7-year-old girl develops breasts and exhibits menstrual bleeding. A 4-cm ovarian cyst is seen on ultrasound. Which of the following is NOT an appropriate action?

  a. estrogen level
  b. birth control pills
  c. GnRH agonists
  d. bone age

5–15. Which of the following is true for premature thelarche?

  a. treat with GnRH agonists
  b. observe
  c. associated with elevated FSH levels
  d. mastectomy

5–16. At which periods of a woman's lifetime are elevated nocturnal LH levels observed?

  a. midpuberty
  b. ovulation
  c. menopause
  d. all of the above

5–17. Which hormone leads to full breast development with rounding of lateral quadrants?

  a. estrogen
  b. progesterone
  c. PRL
  d. all of the above

5–18. Axillary hair usually appears within months or years of pubic hair?

  a. 3 months
  b. 1 year
  c. 2 years
  d. 3 years

5–19. What is the first sign of puberty in males?

  a. pubic hair
  b. voice changes
  c. enlargement of penis
  d. enlargement of testes

5–20. The mean age of initiation of puberty in males is

  a. 9
  b. 11
  c. 13
  d. 15

5–21. Menarche has been shown to occur when body fat reaches

  a. 10 percent
  b. 20 percent
  c. 25 percent
  d. 30 percent

5–22. What is the role of the pineal gland in human puberty?

  a. increases LH secretion
  b. decreases FSH secretion
  c. both a and b
  d. none of the above

5–23. Hypertension may be observed in a phenotypic female with delayed puberty due to

  a. Turner syndrome
  b. 3β-hydroxysteroid dehydrogenase deficiency
  c. 17α-hydroxylase deficiency
  d. all of the above

5–24. Lack of smell and delayed puberty is known as which syndrome?

  a. Kaufman
  b. DeMorsier
  c. Addison
  d. none of the above

5–25. Which of the following clinical features may be seen in women with premature ovarian failure due to immunologic causes?

   a. increased FSH
   b. infertility
   c. vitiligo
   d. all of the above

5–26. Acanthosis nigricans is associated with all of the following EXCEPT

   a. androgen excess
   b. polycystic ovary syndrome (PCOS)

   c. hyperthyroidism
   d. diabetes mellitus type II

5–27. Which of the following is associated with hot flushes?

   a. gonadal dysgenesis
   b. GnRH agonists
   c. hypothalamic amenorrhea
   d. all of the above

Chapter 6

NORMAL AND ABNORMAL SEXUAL DEVELOPMENT

CASE REPORT

A 16-year-old phenotypic female was referred for evaluation of primary amenorrhea. Her rate of growth and development was normal. Breast development occurred at age 10, but the subject failed to develop axillary or pubic hair and had never menstruated.

She denied any significant medical or surgical history. She had not taken any hormonal medication. She had one normal female sibling who was 22 and had a history of normal menstrual cycles.

The physical examination revealed her to be 5'6" in height, 120 lb, and with normal vital signs. Breast development was Tanner stage IV, and no pubic or axillary hair was detected (Fig 6–1). The pelvic exam revealed a short, 3-cm, blind-ending vagina, and a uterus not palpated by rectal exam.

Laboratory testing revealed a follicle-stimulating hormone (FSH) level of 12 mIU, a luteinizing hormone (LH) level of 37 mIU, and a testosterone level of 4.3 ng/ml. A chromosome analysis was obtained, which revealed a 46,XY karyotype (Fig 6–2). The patient was told that she had abnormal gonads with a high chance of malignancy and that they needed to be removed. The patient underwent a laparoscopic orchiectomy and two normal appearing testes were removed. Histologic examination revealed small seminiferous tubules, absent spermatogenesis, and Leydig cell hyperplasia (Fig 6–3). There was no evidence of malignancy at the time of surgery or by histologic examination. No evidence of hernia was detected.

Postoperatively, the patient was started on estrogen therapy, 1.25 mg Premarin every day. When she desires sexual relations, an attempt at di-

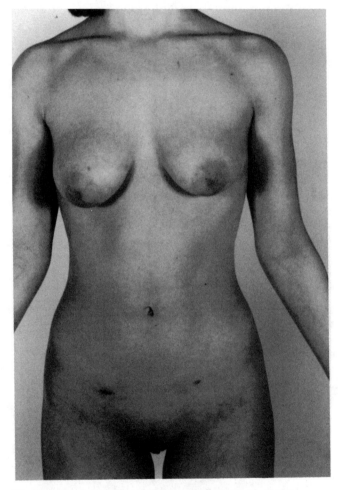

Figure 6–1. Photograph of subject with testicular feminization. Note breast development and absence of pubic and axillary hair. *(Courtesy of Dr. Karen D. Bradshaw, University of Texas Southwestern Medical Center at Dallas, Dallas, TX.)*

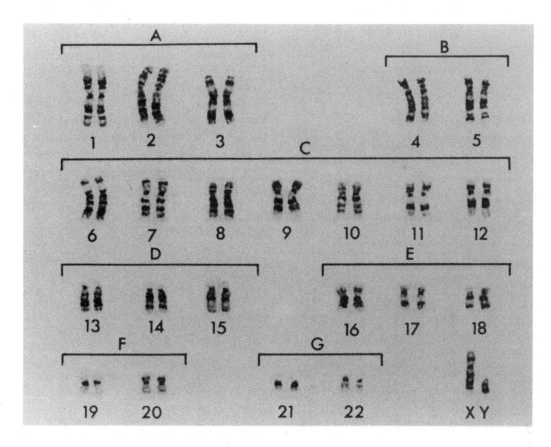

Figure 6–2. Chromosomal analysis of the subject (46,XY).

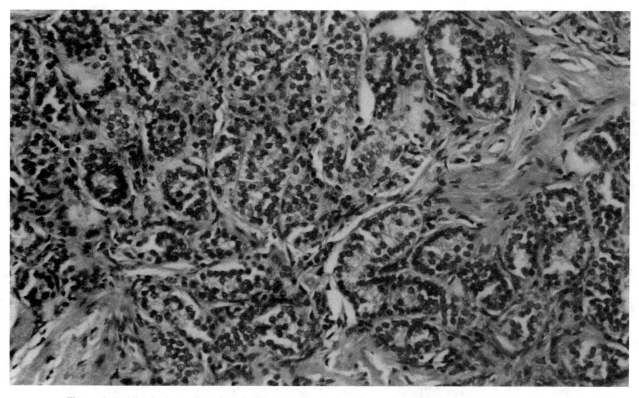

Figure 6–3. Histologic section of testis demonstrating reduced spermatogenesis and Leydig cell hyperplasia. *(Courtesy of Dr. Karen D. Bradshaw, University of Texas Southwestern Medical Center at Dallas, Dallas, TX.)*

lation will be made, but, if unsuccessful, a McIndoe procedure will be offered.

SUMMARY AND CONCLUSIONS

This patient was diagnosed with complete androgen resistance, also known as testicular feminization. In a patient with this disorder (karyotype 46,XY), a defect in androgen action is due to a genetic mutation for the gene for the androgen receptor. A number of mutations for the androgen receptor have been described. Due to androgen resistance, pubic and axillary hair are deficient or absent as in this case. Breast development or gynecomastia occurs because the testes secrete increased amounts of estrogen, and the estrogen receptor is of course normal. The levels of testosterone may be normal, but no androgen effects are detected because of a receptor defect. The uterus is absent because the testes secrete Müllerian-inhibiting substance (MIS). LH values are usually elevated because of androgen insensitivity. FSH levels are normal or elevated. Inguinal hernias are common. Patients with this disorder are raised as females and usually have complete female identity. Because of the risk of malignant gonad transforma-

tion, the testes are removed via laparotomy (Fig 6–4) or laparoscopy. Laparoscopic removal is now the method of choice. The risk for malignancy is very rare prior to age 20, but it is recommended that they be removed after breast development has occurred. Therapy includes estrogen replacement and vaginal dilators or McIndoe vaginoplasty for lengthening the vagina.

BIBLIOGRAPHY

Brown CJ, Goss SJ, Lubahn DB, et al. Androgen receptor locus on the X chromosome: regional localization to Xq11–12 and description of a DNA polymorphism. *Am J Hum Genet.* 44:264k, 1989

Chang C, Kokontis J, Kiao S. Molecular cloning of human and rat complementary DNA encoding androgen receptors. *Science.* 240:324, 1988

DiLauro SD, Behzadian A, Tho SPT, McDonough PG. Probing genomic deoxyribonucleic acid for gene rearrangement in 14 patients with androgen insensitivity syndrome. *Fertil Steril.* 55:481, 1991

Jaffe RB. Disorders of sexual development. In: Yen SSC, Jaffe RB eds. *Reproductive Endocrinology. Physiology, Pathophysiology, and Clinical Management,* 3rd ed. Philadelphia, PA, W. B. Saunders, 1991: 480–510

Lubahn DB, Joseph DR, Sar M, et al. The human androgen receptor: complementary deoxyribonucleic acid cloning, se-

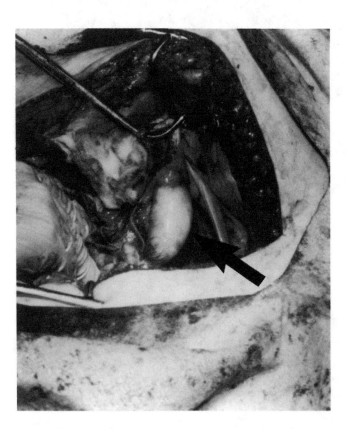

Figure 6–4. Laparotomy demonstrating presence of a testis (see arrow). *(Courtesy of Dr. Karen D. Bradshaw, University of Texas Southwestern Medical Center at Dallas, Dallas, TX.)*

quence analysis, and gene expression in prostate. *Mol Endocrinol.* 2:1265, 1988

Lubahn DB, Joseph DR, Sullivan PM, et al. Cloning of the human androgen receptor complementary DNA and localization to the X chromosome. *Science.* 240:327, 1988

McKusick V. Testicular feminization syndrome (313700). *Mendelian Inheritance in Man* [on line]. October 14, 1991

Morris JM. The syndrome of testicular feminization in male pseudohermaphrodites. *Am J Obstet Gynecol.* 65:1192, 1953

Pereira RR, Brinkmann AO, Ring D, Hodgins MB. Partial androgen insensitivity as a cause of genital maldevelopment. *Helv Paediat Acta.* 39:255, 1984

Tilley WD, Marcelli M, Wilson JD, McPhaul MJ. Characterization and expression of a cDNA encoding the human androgen receptor. *Proc Natl Acad Sci USA.* 86:327, 1989

QUESTIONS

6–1. Which of the following cell types secrete Müllerian-inhibiting hormone?

 a. germinal epithelium
 b. Sertoli cells
 c. Leydig cells
 d. thecal cells

6–2. The gene for the H-Y antigen is found in which chromosome?

 a. Y chromosome, long arm
 b. Y chromosome, short arm
 c. chromosome 16
 d. X chromosome

6–3. Individuals with deletion of Xp11 to Xq21 have which of the following features?

 a. normal ovaries
 b. tall stature
 c. streak ovaries
 d. secondary amenorrhea

6–4. Vanishing testes syndrome, also known as embryonic testicular regression, presents with which of the following phenotypes at birth?

 a. normal female genitalia
 b. normal male genitalia
 c. sexual ambiguity
 d. all of the above

6–5. Which of the following is NOT characteristic of an individual with 5α-reductase type 2 deficiency?

 a. congenital sexual ambiguity
 b. normal testis

 c. absent prostate
 d. absence of growth of the phallus after puberty

6–6. Which of the following is the principal mechanism that prevents the mother and fetus from virilization during pregnancy?

 a. maternal levels of testosterone decline
 b. sex hormone-binding globulin (SHBG) increases
 c. placental aromatase
 d. granulosa cell aromatase increases

6–7. During fetal development, masculinization of male external genitalia occurs at week

 a. 3
 b. 5
 c. 8
 d. 12

6–8. In an individual with true hermaphroditism, with a testis on one side and an ovary on the other, which of the following is NOT true?

 a. congenital sexual ambiguity
 b. Wolffian structures are present on both sides
 c. Wolffian structures are present only on side of testis
 d. Müllerian structures are present on side of ovary

6–9. Which of the following is NOT true about Müllerian-inhibiting substances?

 a. glycoprotein
 b. molecular weight is 72 kD
 c. gene on chromosome 19
 d. secreted after 12 weeks

6–10. Which of the following is the correct sequence of development of the Müllerian system?

 a. elongation, canalization, fusion, septal resorption
 b. elongation, fusion, canalization, septal resorption
 c. septal resorption, elongation, fusion, canalization
 d. septal resorption, fusion, elongation, canalization

6–11. Müllerian and renal anomalies are inherited by which mechanism?

    a. autosomal dominant
    b. autosomal recessive
    c. X-linked
    d. none of the above

6–12. Which of the following is NOT characteristic of the fragile X syndrome?

    a. normal fertility in men
    b. small testes
    c. enlarged testes
    d. X-linked recessive disorder

6–13. Which of the following is NOT characteristic of cryptorchidism?

    a. present in 3 to 4 percent of newborns
    b. bilateral in 75 percent
    c. human chorionic gonadotropin (hCG) used for treatment
    d. increased risk of tumors

6–14. Which of the following tests can be useful in delineating the presence of a uterus in a newborn with sexual ambiguity?

    a. rectal exam
    b. sonogram
    c. genital sinogram
    d. all of the above

6–15. Which of the following is NOT associated with female pseudohermaphroditism?

    a. 46,XX
    b. 5α-reductase deficiency
    c. 21-hydroxylase deficiency
    d. normal Müllerian structures

6–16. MIS deficiency is associated with

    a. normal males
    b. normal females
    c. absence of uterus in a 46,XY male
    d. mental retardation

6–17. In a female with gonadal dysgenesis and absence of secondary sexual characteristics, which of the following is the initial ideal hormone replacement?

    a. low-dose oral contraceptives
    b. 0.3 mg conjugated estrogens
    c. 1.25 mg conjugated estrogens
    d. 0.625 mg conjugated estrogens, plus cyclic progestins

6–18. What is the initial test to be obtained in a 16-year-old female with absence of breast development and immature but normal genitalia?

    a. chromosomes
    b. β-hCG
    c. prolactin
    d. FSH

6–19. Which of the following can be associated with the absence of a uterus?

    a. 46,XX
    b. 46,XY
    c. 5α-reductase
    d. all of the above

6–20. Which of the following is NOT indicated in a child born with congenital sexual ambiguity?

    a. chromosomes
    b. 17-hydroxyprogesterone
    c. FSH
    d. ultrasonography

6–21. Which of the following portions of the Y chromosome is considered the source of the testis development?

    a. TDF
    b. SRY
    c. ZFF
    d. all of the above

6–22. The location of the X-inactivation center has been mapped to which chromosome loci?

    a. Xq15
    b. Xq13
    c. Xq17
    d. none of the above

6–23. Female genitalia are present at birth in which of the following?

    a. presence of one ovary
    b. presence of no ovaries
    c. 17 α-hydroxylase
    d. all of the above

6–24. In which of the following organs or tissues does dihydrotestosterone (DHT) play a greater role than testosterone in masculinization?

    a. penis
    b. muscle
    c. prostate
    d. Wolffian duct

6–25. Which of the following pairs are homologous structures in males and females?

    a. urethral folds–labia majora
    b. clitoris–genital tubercle
    c. labia minora–scrotum
    d. none of the above

6–26. Which of the following is NOT characteristic of Müllerian dysgenesis?

    a. absence of ovaries
    b. high testosterone levels
    c. normal vagina
    d. none of the above

6–27. What is the prevalence of cryptorchidism in term male infants?

    a. 0.5 percent
    b. 1 percent
    c. 10 percent
    d. none of the above

6–28. Characteristics of hypospadias include which of the following?

    a. occurs in 0.8 percent of males
    b. associated with androgen receptor defects
    c. most cases are familial
    d. all of the above

6–29. At which age should clitoral reduction in a female newborn be performed?

    a. immediate newborn period
    b. 3 months
    c. 1 year
    d. puberty

6–30. Which of the following causes of androgen exposure usually causes masculinization of the female genitalia?

    a. norgestimate
    b. aromatase deficiency
    c. hyperreactio luteinalis
    d. all of the above

II

MECHANISMS AND ASSESSMENT OF REPRODUCTIVE HORMONES

Chapter 7

THE MOLECULAR BASIS OF HORMONE ACTION

7–1. Which of the following do NOT exhibit receptors primarily on the cell surface?

   a. peptide hormones
   b. neurotransmitters
   c. steroid hormones
   d. prostaglandins

7–2. Which of the following defines an autocrine substance?

   a. acts on cell type where produced
   b. acts on adjacent cells
   c. acts on distal target cells
   d. all of the above

7–3. Hormones are present in the circulation in concentrations of

   a. 10^{-3} to 10^{-5} mol/L
   b. 10^{-5} to 10^{-7} mol/L
   c. 10^{-7} to 10^{-9} mol/L
   d. 10^{-9} to 10^{-11} mol/L

7–4. The affinity of a hormone for its receptor is defined as

   a. K_d
   b. K_r
   c. K_m
   d. K_w

7–5. In Leydig cells, what percentage of the receptors are unoccupied or spare?

   a. 1 percent
   b. 25 percent
   c. 75 percent
   d. 99 percent

7–6. When the number of cellular spare receptors is reduced from 75 percent to 12 percent, which of the following is true?

   a. The cell is more responsive to a hormone.
   b. The cell is less responsive to a hormone.
   c. The cell response doesn't change.
   d. none of the above

7–7. Which of the following hormones exhibits binding to a seven-transmembrane-domain receptor?

   a. luteinizing hormone (LH)
   b. gonadotropin-releasing hormone (GnRH)
   c. adrenocorticotropic hormone (ACTH)
   d. all of the above

7–8. Which of the following is NOT a component of adenylate cyclase?

   a. G_s
   b. catalytic component
   c. G_r
   d. G_i

7–9. Cholera toxin does NOT exhibit which of the following effects on adenylate cyclase?

   a. catalyzes adenosine diphosphate (ADP) ribosylation of $G_s\alpha$
   b. stimulates ADP ribosylation of $G_s\beta$
   c. permanently activates adenylate cyclase
   d. inhibits glutamyl transpeptidase (GTPase) activity

7–10. Which of the following hormones decreases cyclic adenosine monophosphate (cAMP) levels?

a. LH
b. norepinephrine
c. substance P
d. glucagon

7–11. Which of the following hormones is believed to activate protein kinase C?

a. corticotropin-releasing hormone (CRH)
b. angiotensin II
c. thyroid-stimulating hormone (TSH)
d. substance D

7–12. Which of the following hormones binds to receptors that contain a protein tyrosine kinase domain?

a. epidermal growth factor (EGF)
b. insulin-like growth factor I (IGF-I)
c. transforming growth factor-beta (TGF-β)
d. a and b

7–13. Which of the following hormones activates soluble guanylate cyclase?

a. atrial natriuretic peptide (ANP)
b. nitric oxide (NO)
c. brain atrial natiuretic peptide (BNP)
d. vasopressin

7–14. Which of the following receptors contains a serine/threonine kinase?

a. activin
b. IGF-I
c. TGF-α
d. TSH

7–15. Endocrinopathies due to a gene defect in signal transduction for the estrogen receptor exhibit all of the following EXCEPT

a. tall stature
b. osteoporosis
c. hypogonadism
d. gynecomastia

7–16. Which of the following best describes the term *paracrine?*

a. hormonal effect on distal cells
b. hormonal effect on same cells where produced
c. hormonal effect on pancreatic β cells
d. none of the above

7–17. Which of the following hormones exhibits primary effect on nuclear receptors?

a. LH
b. estrogen
c. hCG
d. all of the above

7–18. Which of the following best defines receptor specificity?

a. low receptor content
b. greater affinity for one biologically active hormone
c. high receptor content
d. lesser affinity for one biologically active hormone

7–19. Which of the following describes the ability of a hormone or substance that prevents full binding of a native hormone but is less biologically active?

a. antagonist
b. competitive antagonist
c. partial agonist
d. super agonist

7–20. Which of the following is true if the number of cell surface receptors are reduced without a change in K_d?

a. binding response curve reduced
b. biological response curve reduced
c. curves remain superimposable
d. all of the above

7–21. Which is true regarding a receptor with seven transmembrane domains?

a. contains four extracellular loops
b. amino half contains transmembrane domains
c. contains three cytoplasmic loops
d. carboxy portion greater in size than amino portion

7–22. Which of the following hormones increases cAMP levels?

  a. substance P
  b. acetylcholine
  c. vasoactive intestinal peptide (VIP)
  d. all of the above

7–23. Which of the following hormones has cell surface receptors that contain primarily tyrosine kinase?

  a. tumor necrosis factor-alpha (TNF-α)
  b. growth hormone (GH)
  c. interleukin-1 beta (IL-1β)
  d. epidermal growth factor (EGF)

7–24. Which of the following receptors when bound to its ligand serves to stimulate endocytosis and removal of receptor and ligand?

  a. ACTH
  b. CRH
  c. low-density lipoprotein (LDL)
  d. none of the above

7–25. Which of the following are subunits of the G_s component of adenylate cyclase?

  a. β_s
  b. β
  c. k
  d. all of the above

7–26. cAMP-dependent protein kinase consists of all of the following EXCEPT

  a. regulatory (R) subunit
  b. R dimers bind four molecules of cAMP
  c. three catalytic (C) units
  d. C subunits free of R express protein kinase activity

7–27. P_{450} enzymes include all of the following EXCEPT

  a. cholesterol side-chain cleavage
  b. aromatase
  c. 17β-hydroxysteroid dehydrogenase
  d. 17α-hydroxylase

LABORATORY ASSESSMENT OF REPRODUCTIVE HORMONES

8–1. Progesterone was isolated in what year?

    a. 1910
    b. 1923
    c. 1941
    d. 1950

8–2. Which of the following hormones can be measured in urine?

    a. 17-ketosteroids
    b. 17-ketogenic steroids
    c. 17-hydroxycorticosteroids
    d. all of the above

8–3. Radioimmunoassay for insulin was developed by

    a. Corner
    b. Zimmerman
    c. Yalow and Berson
    d. Pierce

8–4. The most common isotope used to label proteins is

    a. iodine^{131}
    b. iodine^{125}
    c. phosphorus^{32}
    d. tritium

8–5. The principal advantage of nonradiolabeled procedures is

    a. they are less expensive
    b. they are easier to perform

    c. there is no disposal of radiolabeled compounds
    d. they are faster

8–6. Examples of nonlabeled assays include

    a. fluoroimmunoassays
    b. bioluminescence
    c. chemiluminescence
    d. all of the above

8–7. Which form of prolactin can be measured in the typical pathology laboratory?

    a. big prolactin
    b. big big prolactin
    c. monomeric prolactin
    d. glycosylated prolactin

8–8. Which of the following methods may be used in the future for the real-time measurement of hormone levels?

    a. radioimmunoassay
    b. chemiluminescence assay
    c. bioluminescence assay
    d. amperometric sensors

8–9. Which of the following is NOT a desirable feature of an antiserum?

    a. low equilibrium constant
    b. high specificity
    c. ability to dilute
    d. stability while frozen

8–10. Which of the following is not an advantage of a monoclonal antibody with respect to a polyclonal?

   a. They furnish an indefinite supply of antibody.
   b. They produce highly specific antibodies predictably.
   c. They can produce large quantities of antibody serum.
   d. They are less expensive to produce.

8–11. Which of the following compounds is likely to produce the highest antibody titer as a result of immunization?

   a. thyrotropin-releasing hormone (TRH)
   b. gonadotropin-releasing hormone (GnRH)
   c. follicle-stimulating hormone (FSH)
   d. human chorionic gonadotropin (hCG)

8–12. The most important feature used to select an antiserum is

   a. titer
   b. sensitivity
   c. specificity
   d. affinity

8–13. Which of the following is true regarding reference preparations?

   a. The original standards were produced by the World Health Organization and the National Institutes of Health.
   b. They are available in limited quantity.
   c. These materials were referenced against the bioassays.
   d. all of the above

8–14. The method most frequently used to separate bound from free hormone is

   a. charcoal
   b. immunobead
   c. solid-phase technique
   d. second antibody

8–15. The principal error that can be introduced when using a logit log plot to analyze data is

   a. overestimation of all values
   b. underestimation of all values

   c. underestimation of values at the center of the curve
   d. inaccurate measurement of values inside of the range 15 percent to 85 percent binding

8–16. 17-Hydrocorticosteroids are measured in urine by the

   a. Porter–Silber reaction
   b. Zimmerman reaction
   c. reverse hemolytic plaque assay
   d. metyrapone test

8–17. The term *binding assay* is applied to

   a. radioimmunoassay
   b. enzyme immunoassay
   c. enzyme-linked immunosorbent assay
   d. all of the above

8–18. Which of the following is a disadvantage of urinary nonradiolabeled assay procedures?

   a. expense
   b. need to obtain a 24-hr urinary sample
   c. frequently requires extraction
   d. all of the above

8–19. In the classic binding assay reaction, K_1 and K_3 represent

   a. dissociation of rate constants
   b. association of rate constants
   c. a concentration of bound hormone
   d. concentration of trace

8–20. In the classic binding assay equation, B represents

   a. antibody
   b. trace
   c. hormone concentration
   d. bound hormone

8–21. Which of the following variables most markedly affects the sensitivity of a radioimmunoassay?

   a. ion concentration
   b. volume
   c. temperature
   d. method of separation

8–22. When animals are immunized to produce polyclonal antibodies, which of the following immunoglobulins is NOT produced within the first 2 months?

　　a. IgG
　　b. IgM
　　c. IgE
　　d. none of the above

8–23. Which of the following is an advantage of using antibodies as binding agents?

　　a. They have high equilibrium constants.
　　b. They can detect small concentrations of hormone.
　　c. They are highly specific.
　　d. all of the above

8–24. Which of the following is a major problem encountered in the production of anti-serum?

　　a. It is difficult to obtain a usable serum.
　　b. The antibody may cross-react with an unwanted hormone or site.
　　c. Serum components may nonspecifically affect antibody binding.
　　d. all of the above

8–25. Which of the following cell types is fused with a myeloma cell to produce monoclonal antibodies?

　　a. spleen
　　b. liver
　　c. bone marrow
　　d. thymus

8–26. Which of the following proteins binds testosterone?

　　a. cortisol-binding globulin (CBG)
　　b. sex hormone-binding globulin (SHBG)
　　c. thyroxine-binding globulin (TBG)
　　d. none of the above

8–27. Which of the following chemicals has been used to conjugate steroids to proteins?

　　a. hemisuccinate
　　b. chloral carbonate
　　c. oxime
　　d. all of the above

III

REGULATION OF THE ENDOCRINE SYSTEM OF REPRODUCTIVE MEDICINE

9 NEUROENDOCRINOLOGY OF REPRODUCTION

9–1. Blood flow occurs in the hypothalamic pituitary system in the following manner:

   a. antegrade flow
   b. retrograde flow
   c. interlobar flow
   d. all of the above

9–2. The weight of the pituitary gland is

   a. 10 mg
   b. 10.5 g
   c. 100 g
   d. none of the above

9–3. During pregnancy, the pituitary gland

   a. doubles in size
   b. triples in size
   c. quadruples in size
   d. none of the above

9–4. The most common trophic hormone produced by the pituitary gland is

   a. adrenocorticotropic hormone (ACTH)
   b. prolactin (PRL)
   c. thyroid-stimulating hormone (TSH)
   d. luteinizing hormone (LH)

9–5. Which of the following mechanisms is involved in anterior pituitary control?

   a. juxtacrine
   b. paracrine
   c. autocrine
   d. all of the above

9–6. Which of the following hormones is produced by a large cell (15 to 25 mm) that is distributed throughout the anterior pituitary?

   a. LH and follicle-stimulating hormone (FSH)
   b. ACTH
   c. TSH
   d. PRL

9–7. Which of the following hormone pairs is NOT similar in structure?

   a. growth hormone (GH) and PRL
   b. FSH and LH
   c. ACTH and TSH
   d. LH and TSH

9–8. Gonadotropin-releasing hormone (GnRH) is a

   a. tripeptide
   b. tetradecapeptide
   c. decapeptide
   d. heptapeptide

9–9. Continuous administration of GnRH results in

   a. continuous stimulation of gonadotropin secretion
   b. downregulation of gonadotropin secretion
   c. first stimulation, then downregulation of gonadotropin secretion
   d. first downregulation, then stimulation of gonadotropin secretion

9–10. Following ovulation, LH pulse frequency occurs at

   a. 1-hour intervals
   b. 2-hour intervals
   c. 3-hour intervals
   d. 4-hour intervals

9–11. During the follicular phase, GnRH is released in a

   a. low-amplitude, high-frequency pattern
   b. high-frequency, low-amplitude pattern
   c. low-amplitude, low-frequency pattern
   d. high-amplitude, high-frequency pattern

9–12. Which of the following neurotransmitters is involved in GnRH control?

   a. dopamine
   b. norepinephrine
   c. γ-aminobutyric acid (GABA)
   d. all of the above

9–13. Which of the following is NOT an opiate?

   a. endorphin
   b. enkephalin
   c. prodynorphin
   d. β-lipotropin

9–14. Calmodulin is involved in the regulation of

   a. potassium
   b. sodium
   c. calcium
   d. magnesium

9–15. Which of the following second messengers is associated with GnRH action?

   a. calmodulin
   b. inositol phosphate
   c. tyrosine kinase
   d. all of the above

9–16. Galanin contains how many amino acids?

   a. 3
   b. 10
   c. 29
   d. 39

9–17. Which of the following is a major regulator of blood flow?

   a. serotonin
   b. GABA
   c. nitric oxide (NO)
   d. leptin

9–18. Which investigator(s) suggested that the sex center which regulates reproduction might exist in the brain?

   a. Harris
   b. Markee
   c. Houssay
   d. Holweg and Junkman

9–19. Which investigator(s) demonstrated in vitro that the brain controls ACTH secretion?

   a. Guillemin and Rosenberg
   b. Popa and Fielding
   c. Houssay
   d. Westman and Jacobson

9–20. Guillemin and Shalley won the Nobel prize in 1977 for the structure of

   a. thyrotropin-releasing hormone (TRH)
   b. GnRH
   c. somatostatin
   d. corticotropin-releasing hormone (CRH)

9–21. Circhoral oscillations occur in which area of the brain?

   a. anterior pituitary gland
   b. posterior pituitary gland
   c. arcuate nucleus
   d. amygdala

9–22. Using techniques of electrophysiology and radioimmunoassay, synchronized pulses have been measured which regulate gonadotropin secretion in all of the following compartments EXCEPT the

   a. preoptic area
   b. arcuate nucleus
   c. pituitary portal system
   d. peripheral plasma

9–23. Which of the following peptides interacts with GnRH neurons?

   a. angiotensin-II
   b. neuropeptide-Y
   c. neurotensin
   d. all of the above

9–24. Pro-opiomelantocortin (POMC) is metabolized into which of the following compounds?

   a. ACTH
   b. β-lipotropin
   c. 16-K fragment
   d. all of the above

9–25. Treatment with naloxone causes which of the following in women?

   a. increased frequency and decreased amplitude of LH pulses
   b. decreased frequency and increased amplitude of LH pulses
   c. increased frequency and increased amplitude of LH pulses
   d. decreased frequency and decreased amplitude of LH pulses

9–26. Which of the following is true regarding GnRH action?

   a. GnRH interacts with a population of high-affinity, low-capacity receptors.
   b. GnRH interacts with a population of high-capacity, low-affinity receptors.

   c. GnRH demonstrates self-priming in vivo and in vitro.
   d. all of the above

9–27. GnRH antagonist treatment causes a(n)

   a. decrease in α- and β-chain secretion
   b. decrease in β-chain secretion only
   c. decrease in α-chain secretion only
   d. increase in α- and β-chain secretion

9–28. Which of the following compounds has been shown to directly interact with the GnRH gene?

   a. glucocorticoids
   b. thyroxine
   c. GH
   d. testosterone

9–29. Analysis of the sequence of the GnRH receptor has demonstrated which of the following?

   a. It does not have a transmembrane topology similar to other G-protein couple seven-transmembrane receptors.
   b. Its messenger RNA has been shown to be expressed in the liver and spleen.
   c. There are no differences in binding affinity when tested in different animal model systems.
   d. There is at least a 4-kD difference in molecular size between human and animal models.

Chapter 10

HORMONAL REGULATION OF BREAST PHYSIOLOGY

10–1. Which of the following hormones affects maternal behavior?

   a. progesterone
   b. estradiol
   c. prolactin (PRL)
   d. all of the above

10–2. The administration of gonadotropin-releasing hormone (GnRH) to amenorrheic, lactating, postpartum women results in

   a. stimulation of folliculogenesis
   b. ovulation
   c. normal luteal function
   d. all of the above

10–3. Which of the following syndromes is associated with persistent lactation and an antecedent pregnancy?

   a. Forbes–Albright
   b. Argonz–Del Castillo
   c. Chiari–Frommel
   d. Sheehan

10–4. Which of the following hormones is primarily involved in milk extrusion?

   a. thyrotropin-releasing hormone (TRH)
   b. vasopressin
   c. oxytocin
   d. PRL

10–5. Which of the following hormones is an absolute requisite for mammary development?

   a. cortisol
   b. insulin
   c. progesterone
   d. PRL

10–6. Milk ejection occurs on which day postpartum?

   a. day of delivery
   b. day 1
   c. day 3
   d. day 7

10–7. Milk contains which of the following components?

   a. lactose
   b. proteins
   c. immunoglobulin
   d. all of the above

10–8. The PRL gene is located on which chromosome?

   a. 2
   b. 4
   c. 6
   d. 21

10–9. Which former prolactin has the greatest biological activity?

   a. big prolactin
   b. monomeric prolactin
   c. iso-B prolactin
   d. glycolated prolactin

10–10. Which of the following agents inhibits PRL secretion?

   a. γ-aminobutyric acid (GABA)
   b. TRH
   c. vasoactive intestinal peptide (VIP)
   d. angiotensin-II

10–11. Which of the following agents stimulates PRL secretion?

   a. substance P
   b. histamine
   c. serotonin
   d. all of the above

10–12. Oxytocin is what type of peptide?

   a. tripeptide
   b. decapeptide
   c. undecapeptide
   d. octapeptide

10–13. Suckling results in an elevation in PRL in

   a. 10 minutes
   b. 20 minutes
   c. 30 minutes
   d. 40 minutes

10–14. What percentage of patients ovulate and menstruate by 6 months postpartum?

   a. 10 percent
   b. 20 percent
   c. 30 percent
   d. 40 percent

10–15. Which of the following syndromes is associated with lactation and the presence of a pituitary tumor?

   a. Forbes–Albright
   b. Argonz–Del Castillo
   c. Chiari–Frommel
   d. Sheehan

10–16. Long-term treatment with which of the following hormones prevents the diurnal change in lactotrope proliferation?

   a. progesterone
   b. estradiol
   c. PRL
   d. cortisol

10–17. Which of the following hormones has been shown to influence nursing behavior?

   a. progesterone
   b. estradiol
   c. PRL
   d. all of the above

10–18. Which of the following mechanisms is involved in maintenance of postpartum amenorrhea?

   a. reduced GnRH secretion
   b. lack of responsiveness of pituitary gonadotrope to GnRH
   c. PRL suppression of granulosa cell growth
   d. none of the above

10–19. Which of the following compounds has been associated with the involution of the lactating mammary gland?

   a. cortisol
   b. thyroxine
   c. insulin-like growth factor (IGF)
   d. growth hormone (GH)

10–20. Which of the following hormones stimulates duct development in the breast?

   a. progesterone
   b. estradiol
   c. GH
   d. PRL

10–21. "Witch's milk," which is expressible from the nipples of some newborn girls, is caused by

   a. progesterone production
   b. estradiol production
   c. increase in fetal PRL
   d. increase in fetal cortisol

10–22. The human leukocyte antigen (HLA) is located on chromosome 6 near the gene for

    a. GH
    b. adrenocorticotropic hormone (ACTH)
    c. PRL
    d. follicle-stimulating hormone (FSH)

10–23. The lactotrope makes up what percentage of the pituitary cell population?

    a. 10 percent
    b. 20 percent
    c. 30 percent
    d. 40 percent

10–24. What is the molecular weight of monomeric PRL?

    a. 22,000
    b. 50,000
    c. 100,000
    d. 25,000

10–25. PRL contains what number of amino acids?

    a. 10
    b. 39
    c. 198
    d. 13

10–26. Infusion of which of the following compounds increases PRL secretion?

    a. TRH
    b. L-dopa
    c. arginine
    d. all of the above

THE OVARY

11–1. During which week of fetal life do the primordial germ cells migrate from the yolk sac to the site of the future gonad?

    a. 3
    b. 6
    c. 9
    d. 12

11–2. At which week of fetal life can the ovary be histologically identified?

    a. 4
    b. 6
    c. 8
    d. 10

11–3. At which stage of meiosis does the oocyte arrest during fetal life?

    a. pachytene
    b. leptotene
    c. diplotene
    d. zygotene

11–4. Which of the following enzymes is missing in the fetal ovary?

    a. aromatase
    b. 17α-hydroxylase
    c. both of the above
    d. none of the above

11–5. Which of the following substances stimulates Wolffian duct development?

    a. Müllerian-inhibiting substance (MIS)
    b. testosterone
    c. dehydroepiandrosterone sulfate (DHEAS)
    d. dihydrotestosterone (DHT)

11–6. When is the follicle-stimulating hormone/luteinizing hormone (FSH/LH) ratio <1?

    a. fetal life at 20 wk
    b. postnatal at 3 mo

    c. reproductive years
    d. menopause

11–7. Which of the following is true concerning human granulosa cells?

    a. They exhibit high levels of aromatase.
    b. They have a direct blood supply.
    c. They exhibit high levels of 17α-hydroxylase.
    d. all of the above

11–8. The mechanisms of atresia include which of the following?

    a. decline in circulatory FSH levels
    b. decline in circulatory estradiol levels
    c. apoptosis
    d. none of the above

11–9. The oocyte maintains linear growth until which stage of development?

    a. primary
    b. secondary
    c. tertiary
    d. graafian

11–10. Secondary interstitial cells are derived from

    a. primary interstitial cells
    b. contractile cells
    c. atretic follicles
    d. none of the above

11–11. The hilum of the ovary does NOT contain

    a. Call–Exner bodies
    b. crystalloids of Reinke
    c. hilus cells
    d. androgens

11–12. Which of the following is NOT true regarding corpus luteum development following ovulation?

   a. Proliferation occurs on day 1.
   b. Capillary invasion is initiated on day 4.
   c. Fibroblasts appear in the antral cavity on day 5.
   d. Maximal capillary development occurs on day 8.

11–13. All of the following hormones stimulate luteinizing hormone-releasing hormone (LHRH) release EXCEPT

   a. serotonin
   b. epinephrine
   c. norepinephrine
   d. estradiol

11–14. Circhoral is

   a. low-grade frequency changes every 30 days
   b. intermittent frequency changes every 24 hours
   c. high-frequency changes every hour
   d. none of the above

11–15. Which of the following hormones inhibits FSH release?

   a. progesterone
   b. inhibin
   c. follistatin
   d. all of the above

11–16. Which of the following represents the primary source of cholesterol for progestin secretion by the human corpus luteum?

   a. very low-density lipoprotein (VLDL)
   b. high-density lipoprotein 2 (HDL2)
   c. HDL
   d. LDL

11–17. Which of the following enzymes is the rate-limiting step in steroid synthesis of hormones?

   a. aromatase
   b. 17α-hydroxylase
   c. 17/20 desmolase
   d. cholesterol side-chain cleavage

11–18. Which type of 17β-hydroxysteroid dehydrogenase (17β-HSD) is found in highest quantities in human granulosa cells?

   a. type I
   b. type II
   c. type III
   d. type IV

11–19. Which of the following enzymes is localized primarily in the theca interna cells of the follicle?

   a. $P_{450_{AROM}}$
   b. $P_{450_{17\alpha}}$
   c. 17β-HSD type III
   d. none of the above

11–20. The estrogen receptor consists of all of the following EXCEPT

   a. carboxy terminus hinge region
   b. deoxyribonucleic acid (DNA)-binding domain
   c. a transcriptional activation of functional domain at the nitrogen terminus
   d. steroid response elements

11–21. How many germ cells are present in the ovary at birth?

   a. 8 million
   b. 1 million
   c. 500,000
   d. 450,000

11–22. Which of the following cell types produce oocyte maturation inhibitor which inhibits meiosis in utero?

   a. oocyte
   b. theca externa
   c. granulosa
   d. none of the above

11–23. During puberty, which of the following is NOT true?

   a. LH > FSH
   b. FSH > LH
   c. inhibin increases
   d. none of the above

11–24. Which of the following is NOT true regarding the prepubertal state (ie, 6-year-old female)?

    a. GnRH pulses are low or absent.

    b. Exogenous therapy with GnRH given in pulses will not induce puberty.

    c. LH and FSH levels are low in 45,X individuals.

    d. Estrogen levels are low.

11–25. Which of the following enzymes exhibit decreased expression in the reticularis following adrenarche?

    a. aromatase

    b. 17β-HSD type 1

    c. 3β-HSD

    d. cytochrome P$_{450_{scc}}$

11–26. Adrenarche is delayed in which of the following?

    a. Kallmann syndrome

    b. gonadal dysgenesis

    c. 21-hydroxylase deficiency

    d. none of the above

11–27. Which of the following is NOT true regarding inhibin?

    a. secreted in three forms: A, B, C

    b. molecular weight 32,000

    c. secreted by granulosa cells

    d. related to transforming growth factor-beta (TGF-β)

11–28. Which of the following describes the mechanism of lack of growth in African pygmies?

    a. low growth hormone (GH) levels

    b. absence of GH receptor

    c. low insulin-like growth factor I (IGF-I) levels

    d. all of the above

11–29. Which of the following nonsteroidal factors is produced by the ovary?

    a. oxytocin

    b. relaxin

    c. transforming growth factor-alpha (TGF-α)

    d. all of the above

11–30. Trigintan describes which of the following?

    a. low-frequency changes of gonadotropin which occur every 30 days

    b. changes of gonadotropins every 24 hours

    c. high-frequency changes which occur every hour

    d. none of the above

11–31. Which of the following enzymes is NOT expressed in granulosa cells?

    a. P$_{450_{scc}}$

    b. aromatase

    c. 3β-HSD

    d. none of the above

11–32. The production rate of a hormone is which of the following?

    a. MCR (metabolic clearance rate) $\times$ SR (secretion rate)

    b. MCR $\div$ concentration

    c. MCR + concentration

    d. MCR $\times$ concentration

Chapter 12

THE NORMAL MENSTRUAL CYCLE: THE COORDINATED EVENTS OF THE HYPOTHALAMIC–PITUITARY–OVARIAN AXIS AND THE FEMALE REPRODUCTIVE TRACT

12–1. Which of the following is correct regarding the length of the phase of the normal menstrual cycle?

    a. follicular phase usually 14 days
    b. luteal phase usually 14 days
    c. menses lasts 2 days
    d. menses lasts 8 days

12–2. The first phase of follicular growth is initiated by

    a. inhibin
    b. luteal-phase decline in luteinizing hormone (LH)
    c. activin
    d. none of the above

12–3. In women, ovulation occurs on which side compared to the previous cycle?

    a. contralateral
    b. ipsilateral
    c. random
    d. all of the above

12–4. Follicle-stimulating hormone (FSH) levels decline in the midfollicular phase in response to all of the following EXCEPT

    a. inhibin
    b. estrogen
    c. negative feedback mechanisms
    d. activin

12–5. Which of the following is the second stage of follicular development?

    a. recruitment
    b. regression
    c. dominance
    d. none of the above

12–6. FSH receptors are located in

    a. thecal cells
    b. thecal–luteal cells
    c. granulosa cells
    d. all of the above

12–7. Which of the following is NOT true?

    a. FSH induces aromatase.
    b. FSH induces estrogen secretion.

c. FSH plus testosterone induces LH release.

d. FSH plus estrogen induces LH receptors.

12–8. Small antral follicles secrete primarily

a. estrogen
b. testosterone
c. progesterone
d. dehydroepiandrosterone (DHEA)

12–9. The concentration of estrogen in follicular fluid is

a. less than circulatory levels
b. equal to circulatory levels
c. absent
d. greater than circulatory levels

12–10. During the menstrual cycle

a. FSH levels decline prior to ovulation
b. FSH levels rise during ovulation
c. LH levels rise prior to ovulation
d. all of the above

12–11. The peak of LH secretion precedes ovulation by how many hours?

a. 36
b. 10 to 16
c. 24
d. 8 to 10

12–12. Which of the following is NOT true regarding the process of ovulation?

a. Follicular pressure increases.
b. Prostaglandin E increases.
c. Prostaglandin F increases.
d. Hydroxyeicosatetraeonic and methyl esters (HETES) increase.

12–13. The effect of indomethacin on ovulation is

a. no effect
b. inhibition
c. stimulation
d. delays

12–14. The levels of inhibin at the time of ovulation

a. decrease
b. increase markedly

c. increase modestly
d. are unchanged

12–15. Which of the following is NOT true regarding the dating of the endometrium?

a. Glandular mitoses are high during the proliferative phase.
b. Pseudostratification of nuclei occurs during the proliferative phase.
c. Stromal edema occurs during the proliferative phase.
d. Pseudodecidual reaction occurs during the proliferative phase.

12–16. At which time of reproductive life are anovulatory cycles common?

a. immediately after puberty
b. prior to menopause
c. during episodes of stress
d. all of the above

12–17. At the end of the luteal phase

a. activin increases
b. FSH increases
c. estrone levels increase
d. none of the above

12–18. The selection stage of follicular development occurs during which days of the menstrual cycle?

a. 1 to 3
b. 3 to 5
c. 5 to 7
d. 7 to 9

12–19. Which of the following is found in follicular fluid?

a. prolactin (PRL)
b. vasopressin
c. estrone
d. all of the above

12–20. Which of the following hormones is found in high concentration in follicular fluid of large follicles?

a. testosterone
b. PRL
c. progesterone
d. none of the above

12–21. Which of the following hormones primes the hypothalamus to release gonadotropin-releasing hormone (GnRH) or luteinizing hormone-releasing hormone (LHRH)?

   a. estrogen
   b. progesterone
   c. LH
   d. activin

12–22. During the early part of the proliferative phase, LH pulse frequencies occur at

   a. 30 seconds
   b. 30 minutes
   c. 60 minutes
   d. 2 hours

12–23. The first polar body release is associated with which of the following?

   a. in utero at 20 weeks
   b. following FSH surge
   c. second stage of meiosis
   d. none of the above

12–24. Which of the following is true regarding estradiol levels just prior to the peak of LH?

   a. levels fall
   b. levels are unchanged
   c. levels increase
   d. all of the above

12–25. Which of the following is NOT important in control of steroid production by the human corpus luteum?

   a. LH secretory patterns
   b. LH receptor content
   c. cholesterol formed de novo
   d. low-density lipoprotein (LDL) cholesterol

12–26. A short luteal phase may be due to

   a. poor follicle development
   b. low FSH levels
   c. PRL elevation
   d. all of the above

12–27. Which of the following is involved in luteolysis in women?

   a. renin
   b. angiotensin
   c. oxytocin
   d. all of the above

THE PHYSIOLOGY OF THE TESTIS AND MALE REPRODUCTIVE TRACT AND DISORDERS OF TESTICULAR FUNCTION

CASE REPORT

At age 18, a male was evaluated for delayed sexual development. He had no other complaints. He denied other significant past medical or surgical history or family history.

The physical examination revealed a tall male, 6'3" in height, with a weight of 148 lb (Fig 13–1). His blood pressure was 110/70. There was only fine hair development on his upper lip. Axillary hair was present, but gynecomastia was absent. The examination of the genitalia revealed reduced pubic hair with a female escutcheon. The phallus was small and the testes were reduced in size (left, 4 ml; right, 5 ml).

Laboratory testing revealed increased gonadotropins and a low testosterone level (Table 13–1). A chromosome analysis was obtained and revealed a 47,XXY karyotype.

A diagnosis of Klinefelter syndrome was made, and the subject was placed on testosterone injections every 2 weeks. In the first year of therapy, he noted increased facial hair with beard growth, full male escutcheon, muscle mass, and increased growth of the phallus.

At age 32, he describes adequate sexual function with erections and ejaculations over the past 14 years. However, he has numerous brushes with the law and has spent time in jail where he is currently incarcerated. He receives 200 mg of testosterone cypionate injections every 2 weeks.

SUMMARY AND CONCLUSIONS

The diagnosis of this condition is Klinefelter syndrome, which is a disorder characterized by delayed and impaired sexual maturation and small testes. It is also associated with varying degrees of gynecomastia and azoospermia. This defect is due to an abnormal karyotype associated with an extra X chromosome, most often 47,XXY or occasionally 46,XY/47,XXY (mosaic form). In this individual, the size of the testes and levels of testosterone were not as severely affected as most, explaining in part the absence of gynecomastia. However, social maladjustment was present, which is quite common. Treatment is testosterone injections, and infertility is best treated with donor sperm.

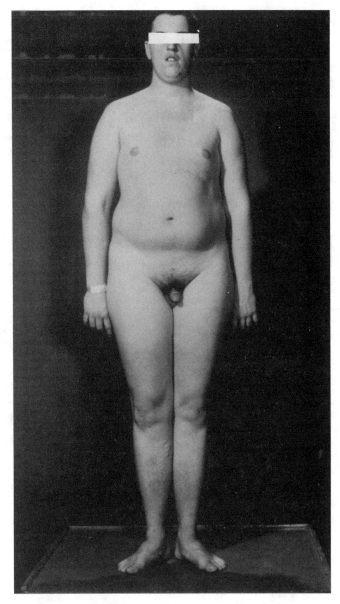

Figure 13–1. Photograph of the subject with 46,XXY Klinefelter syndrome. *(Courtesy of Dr. James Griffin, University of Texas Southwestern Medical Center at Dallas, Dallas, TX.)*

Table 13–1. Gonadotropin and Testosterone Levels

	Klinefelter Patient	Normal Adult Range
LH mIU/ml	62	<15
FSH mIU/ml	82	5–25
Testosterone ng/dL	167	300–1200

BIBLIOGRAPHY

de la Chapelle A. Analytic review: nature and origin of male with XX sex chromosomes. *Am J Human Genet.* 24:71, 1972

Gabrilove JL, Frieberg EK, Nicholis GL. Testicular function in Klinefelter's syndrome. *J Urol.* 124:825, 1980

Gordon DL, Krmpotic E, Thomas W, et al. Pathologic testicular findings in Klinefelter's syndrome. 47,XXY vs 46,XY/47,XXY. *Arch Intern Med.* 130:726, 1972

Nielsen J, Pelsen B. Follow-up 20 years later of 34 Klinefelter males with karyotype 47,XXY and 16 hypogonadal males with karyotype 46,XY. *Human Genet.* 77:188, 1987

Samaan NA, Stepanas AV, Danziger J, et al. Reactive pituitary abnormalities in patients with Klinefelter's and Turner's syndromes. *Arch Intern Med.* 139:198, 1979

Schibler D, Brook CGD, Kind HP, et al. Growth and body proportions in 54 boys and men with Klinefelter's syndrome. *Helv Paediatr Acta.* 29:325, 1974

QUESTIONS

13–1. At which week of fetal development is the testis first identifiable?

    a. 3
    b. 6
    c. 9
    d. 12

13–2. Which of the following is NOT true concerning Leydig cells in the human testis?

    a. Lipid droplets contain esterified cholesterol.
    b. Cholesterol is derived in part from circulating lipoproteins.
    c. Cellular testosterone is high.
    d. Mitochondria are the site of cholesterol side-chain cleavage.

13–3. Which of the following is true concerning the vas deferens?

    a. It is a tubular structure 60 cm in length.
    b. It contains on cross-section an inner circular muscular layer.
    c. The cells lining the lumen do not have cilia.
    d. It begins at the cauda epididymis and terminates near the prostate.

13–4. Luteinizing hormone-releasing hormone (LHRH) stimulates luteinizing hormone (LH) and follicle-stimulating hormone (FSH) release by which of the following mechanisms?

   a. calcium dependent
   b. diacylglycerol dependent
   c. cyclic adenosine monophosphate (cAMP) independent
   d. all of the above

13–5. FSH regulates the synthesis of which of the following in the Sertoli cells?

   a. protein kinase C
   b. aromatase
   c. testosterone-binding globulin (TeBG)
   d. a and b

13–6. Dihydrotestosterone (DHT) has which of the following metabolic consequences?

   a. converts rapidly to testosterone
   b. stimulates Wolffian duct development
   c. converts slowly to 17β-estradiol
   d. none of the above

13–7. Which of the following represents the third enzymatic sequence in the formation of testosterone from cholesterol?

   a. 3β-hydroxysteroid dehydrogenase (3β-HSD)
   b. 17β-HSD (17β-HSOR)
   c. P_{450scc}
   d. $P_{450 17\alpha}$

13–8. Which of the following is true regarding testosterone transportation in blood?

   a. 14 percent free (unbound)
   b. 84 percent bound to TeBG
   c. 54 percent bound to albumin
   d. none of the above

13–9. Which is true regarding 5α-reductase?

   a. There are five types.
   b. Type 1 is expressed in genital skin.
   c. Type 2 is expressed in liver.
   d. all of the above

13–10. Aromatase activity is present in a variety of tissues. Which of the following is true regarding expression in these tissues?

   a. There are three specific types of aromatase.
   b. FSH regulates expression in each tissue.
   c. Expression is determined by the tissue.
   d. The P_{450} enzyme complex in the testis is different than that in the ovary.

13–11. Sperm formation takes approximately how many days?

   a. 30
   b. 50
   c. 70
   d. 90

13–12. The hormonal control of spermatogenesis involves

   a. LH and FSH
   b. FSH alone
   c. inhibin and LH
   d. inhibin and FSH

13–13. Which of the following forms of androgen therapy is the primary choice for hypogonadism?

   a. methyltestosterone
   b. methenolone
   c. testosterone enanthate
   d. testosterone patch

13–14. The first sign of male puberty is which of the following?

   a. pubic hair
   b. increase in penile length
   c. deepening/cracking of voice
   d. testicular enlargement

13–15. The normal range of plasma testosterone in men is

   a. 3 to 10 pg/ml
   b. 3 to 10 μg/ml
   c. 3 to 10 ng/ml
   d. 3 to 10 mg/ml

13–16. Testosterone levels

    a. are highest in the evening
    b. are highest in the morning
    c. are highest at noon
    d. do not exhibit diurnal rhythm

13–17. What is considered the lowest limit of normal for a sperm count?

    a. ≤10 million/ml
    b. ≤20 million/ml
    c. ≤40 million/ml
    d. ≤60 million/ml

13–18. Which of the following is true regarding precocious pseudopuberty in males?

    a. virilization and spermatogenesis occur
    b. virilization only
    c. spermatogenesis only
    d. spermatogenesis precedes virilization

13–19. Isolated gonadotropin deficiency is associated with

    a. Kallmann syndrome
    b. Klinefelter syndrome
    c. autosomal dominance
    d. all of the above

13–20. Hyperprolactinemia is associated with males with

    a. galactorrhea
    b. impotence
    c. normal semen analysis
    d. all of the above

13–21. Klinefelter syndrome is characterized by all of the following EXCEPT

    a. gynecomastia
    b. 47,XXY
    c. normal testicular size
    d. elevated LH levels

13–22. Treatment of Klinefelter syndrome includes

    a. testosterone injections
    b. psychological consulting
    c. donor sperm for fertility
    d. all of the above

13–23. Which of the following characterizes the process of germ migration?

    a. differs in males and females
    b. occurs at 7 weeks' gestation
    c. amoeboid movement
    d. all of the above

13–24. The gubernaculum

    a. is involved in germ cell development
    b. connects inguinal region with the testis
    c. increases length in response to inhibin
    d. all of the above

13–25. Which of the following is involved in testicular descent?

    a. Müllerian-inhibiting substance (MIS)
    b. androgens
    c. intra-abdominal pressure
    d. all of the above

13–26. The central portion of the Wolffian duct develops into the

    a. vas deferens
    b. epididymis
    c. seminal vesicles
    d. prostate

13–27. DHT stimulates growth and development of the

    a. muscle
    b. Wolffian duct
    c. external genitalia
    d. all of the above

13–28. LHRH contains how many peptides?

    a. 3
    b. 9
    c. 10
    d. 11

13–29. Which of the following can induce virilization in prepubertal males?

    a. 17α-hydroxylase
    b. 21-hydroxylase deficiency
    c. aromatase deficiency
    d. Addison's disease

13–30. Leydig cell hyperplasia as a cause of precocious puberty can be treated with all the following EXCEPT

   a. gonadotropin-releasing hormone (GnRH) agonists
   b. testolactone
   c. flutamide
   d. aromatase inhibitors

13–31. Which of the following treatments or diseases is associated with low testosterone levels?

   a. GnRH agonist
   b. acquired immune deficiency syndrome (AIDS)

   c. prednisone
   d. all of the above

13–32. Hernia uteri inguinale is associated with

   a. infertility
   b. elevated LH levels
   c. absence of MIS
   d. all of the above

IV

ABNORMALITIES OF THE ENDOCRINE SYSTEM OF REPRODUCTIVE MEDICINE

Chapter 14

ASSESSMENT OF THE FEMALE PATIENT

14–1. Premature thelarche differs from true precocious puberty in that premature thelarche is associated with

    a. gradual progressive increases in serum estradiol
    b. pubic hair development
    c. both of the above
    d. none of the above

14–2. Puberty is considered delayed in girls if which of the following have not occurred?

    a. breast development by age 13
    b. menarche by age 16
    c. more than 5 years passed from the onset of breast development without menarche
    d. all of the above

14–3. Which of the following are consistent with amenorrhea due to a central origin?

    a. atrophic vagina
    b. galactorrhea
    c. loss of body weight
    d. all of the above

14–4. Which of the following is NOT true regarding height and sexual development?

    a. Estrogen regulates final adult height.
    b. Early sexual development results in shorter adult height.
    c. Testosterone regulates final adult height.
    d. none of the above

14–5. Which of the following is correct regarding arm span?

    a. It is normally 3 inches greater than height.
    b. It is normally 3 inches less than height.

    c. It is normally equal to height.
    d. It has no relation to height.

14–6. A puffy face, thickening of the lips and tongue, and roughening of the skin best describe

    a. Addison's disease
    b. Cushing syndrome
    c. myxedema
    d. panhypopituitarism

14–7. Pallid, hairless, smooth, and dry skin best describes

    a. Addison's disease
    b. Graves' disease
    c. Sheehan syndrome
    d. Albright's disease

14–8. Parabasal cells from the vagina are associated with all of the following EXCEPT

    a. prepuberty
    b. ovulation
    c. menopause
    d. oral contraceptive pills

14–9. A maturation index of 90:5:5 best describes

    a. the proliferative phase
    b. the luteal phase
    c. menopause
    d. none of the above

14–10. Which of the following are the usual medications used to induce withdrawal bleeding?

    a. clomiphene citrate
    b. depo-medroxyprogesterone acetate
    c. ethinyl estradiol
    d. none of the above

14–11. Which of the following sites is composed primarily of trabecular bone?

    a. distal radius
    b. vertebral body
    c. distal femur
    d. proximal femur

14–12. If the serum follicle-stimulating hormone (FSH) levels are elevated in a woman with amenorrhea, which of the following is true?

    a. Laparoscopy is usually indicated.
    b. A prolactin (PRL) level should be obtained.
    c. A luteinizing hormone (LH) level should be obtained.
    d. none of the above

14–13. Which of the following is most likely in a woman with secondary amenorrhea and a low FSH level?

    a. ovarian failure
    b. pregnancy
    c. Müllerian agenesis
    d. none of the above

14–14. Which test is best to confirm acromegaly?

    a. basal growth hormone (GH) level
    b. exercise-induced GH level
    c. somastatin-induced GH level
    d. basal insulin-like growth factor I (IGF-I) level

14–15. An 18-year-old phenotypic female presents with primary amenorrhea, no breast development, absent uterus, and markedly elevated FSH levels. Which of the following is a possible diagnosis?

    a. Müllerian agenesis
    b. testicular feminization

    c. embryonic testicular regression syndrome
    d. all of the above

14–16. All of the following are characteristic of 45,X gonadal dysgenesis EXCEPT

    a. dysplastic toenails
    b. short fourth metacarpals
    c. skin hyperpigmentation
    d. shield-like chest

14–17. Which of the following is NOT characteristic of estrogen production?

    a. ferning of cervical mucus
    b. spinnbarkeit
    c. maturation index of 80:10:10
    d. maturation index of 10:10:80

14–18. Which of the following is suggested in a woman with an elevated dehydroepiandrosterone sulfate (DHEAS) level of 5.0 µg/ml, with hirsutism and 2° amenorrhea?

    a. adrenal virilizing adenoma
    b. polycystic ovary syndrome (PCOS)
    c. adult-onset 21-hydroxylase deficiency
    d. Cushing syndrome

14–19. A low thyroid-stimulating hormone (TSH) level (<0.01 µU/mL) suggests

    a. primary hypothyroidism
    b. hyperthyroidism
    c. hyperprolactinemia
    d. tertiary hypothyroidism

14–20. Which of the following is NOT associated with elevated prolactin (PRL) levels?

    a. empty sella
    b. phenothiazine
    c. oral contraceptives
    d. Depo-Provera

14–21. Which of the following is NOT characteristic of adult-onset adrenal hyperplasia due to 21-hydroxylase deficiency?

    a. elevated cortisol
    b. elevated 17-hydroxyprogesterone
    c. hirsutism
    d. oligomenorrhea

14–22. Cushing syndrome is characterized by which of the following symptoms or signs?

   a. hirsutism
   b. weakness
   c. hypertension
   d. all of the above

14–23. Diabetes insipidus is characterized by

   a. decreased urine output
   b. increased plasma osmolality
   c. delayed onset of labor
   d. none of the above

14–24. A chromosome analysis is indicated in women with primary amenorrhea associated with

   a. galactorrhea
   b. low FSH
   c. elevated FSH
   d. headaches

14–25. All of the following are always surgical indications for Müllerian developmental or acquired defects EXCEPT

   a. transverse vaginal septum
   b. bicornuate uterus
   c. imperforate hymen
   d. Asherman syndrome

14–26. Hirsutism is characterized by increased hair growth in all of the following sites EXCEPT

   a. breasts
   b. face
   c. arms
   d. abdomen

14–27. The evaluation of all secondary amenorrheic women should include all of the following EXCEPT

   a. beta-human chorionic gonadotropin (β-hCG)
   b. FSH
   c. testosterone
   d. PRL

Chapter 15

ANOVULATION OF CNS ORIGIN: ANATOMIC CAUSES

CASE REPORT

The patient is a 17-year-old white female who underwent menarche at 13 years of age. She presented with secondary amenorrhea in May 1978 (15 years of age). She complained of both galactor-rhea and continuous frontal headache. In August 1979, anterior, posterior, and lateral tomograms were found to be negative for the presence of a pituitary tumor. In January 1980, her serum prolactin (PRL) level was found to be 385 ng/ml, reference to National Institutes of Health VLSII standard. A

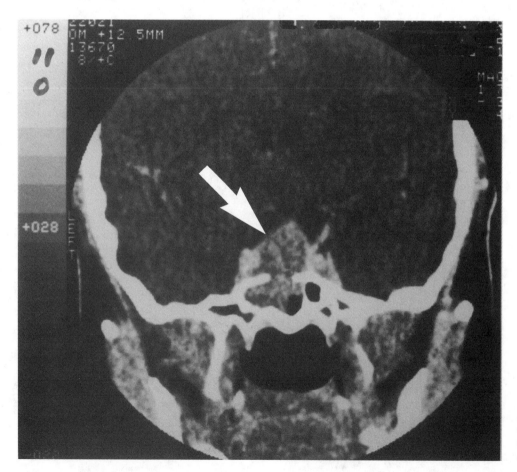

Figure 15–1. CT scan of patient with a prolactin-secreting pituitary macroadenoma. Suprasellar extension is evident.

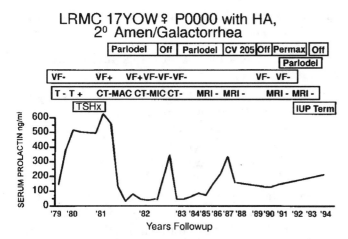

Figure 15–2. Time line of treatment of patient with a pituitary macroadenoma over 15 years.

polytomogram of the sella turcica was also interpreted as negative for the presence of a tumor. In July 1980, a computed axial tomogram (CT) showed an enlarged and full sella turcica. In September 1980, the patient underwent a transsphenoidal hypophysectomy, and the tissue sample was positive for a prolactinoma. By July 1981, the patient's PRL level had increased to 625 ng/ml, and a CT scan was positive for a suprasellar macroadenoma (Fig 15–1). She had persistent headaches and bitemporal hemianopia. By August 1981, her serum PRL level was 572 ng/ml, and she was begun on bromocriptine therapy, 2.5 mg t.i.d. Within a month, her serum PRL level had decreased to 124 ng/ml. After 2 months of therapy, the serum PRL level had decreased to 32 ng/ml (normal, 5 to 30 ng/ml). By February 1982, a CT scan showed the presence of only a small microadenoma, and the bitemporal hemianopia had resolved. Subsequently, the patient has had magnetic resonance imaging (MRI) or CT scans at about 5-year intervals; these continue to show no tumor. She has been treated with bromocriptine (Parlodel), pergolide mesylate (Permax), and norprolac (CV205-502). She has been off medication on three occasions for a year each time. In 1992, she conceived and gave birth to a term infant and was treated with no medication and breast fed thereafter. Subsequently, she has returned to bromocriptine therapy and is doing well today, some 18 years after her initial diagnosis (Fig 15–2).

SUMMARY AND CONCLUSIONS

This case challenges a great deal of the dogma that exists regarding the long-term management of patients with macroadenomas. First of all, this patient responded appropriately to treatment with a first-generation dopamine agonist, as do most individuals. She had a prompt reduction of her serum PRL levels and a marked shrinkage of the size of the pituitary tumor. Further, she was maintained on long-term therapy with no reoccurrence and managed with serum PRL levels and interval history every 6 months, with imaging and visual field examinations being used sparingly. Further, she was able to achieve pregnancy without difficulty, carry the pregnancy to term, and breast feed with no exacerbation of her symptoms. While this represents only a case study, this is the typical response of patients that we have followed, who have been diagnosed during their adolescence and followed for intervals of 15 to 20 years.

BIBLIOGRAPHY

Costello RT. Subclinical adenoma of the pituitary gland. *Am J Pathol.* 12:205, 1936

Kovacs K, Horvath E. Pathology of pituitary tumors. *Endocrinol Metab Clin N Am.* 16:529, 1987

Kwekkeboon DJ, de Jong FH, Lamberts SWJ. Gonadotropin release by clinically nonfunctioning and gonadotroph pituitary adenomas in vivo and in vitro: relation to sex and effects of thyrotropin-releasing hormone, gonadotropin-releasing hormone, and bromocriptine. *J Clin Endocrinol Metab.* 68:1128, 1989

Molitch ME. Pathologic hyperprolactinemia. *Endocrinol Metab Clin N Am.* 21:877, 1991

Molitch ME, Elton RL, Blackwell RE, et al. Bromocriptine as primary therapy for prolactin-secreting macroadenomas: results of a prospective multicenter study. *J Clin Endocrinol Metab.* 60:698, 1985

QUESTIONS

15–1. The World Health Organization adenohypophyseal neoplasm staging system is based on which of the following?

   a. biochemical studies, histology, immunocytochemistry

   b. clinical results and imaging

   c. operative findings and electron microscopic studies

   d. all of the above

15–2. Which of the following best describes the thyroid-stimulating hormone (TSH)-secreting pituitary adenoma?

  a. It is a common cause of hyperthyroidism.
  b. The majority of the tumors are >10 mm.
  c. These tumors are not associated with an elevation in α-subunit level.
  d. The diagnosis is facilitated by the high-sensitivity TSH immunoassay.

15–3. Which of the following is associated with the etiology of pituitary tumors?

  a. defective signal transduction
  b. defective regulation of dopamine metabolism
  c. development of aberrant blood supply
  d. all of the above

15–4. Which of the following is the most common presenting complaint associated with prolactinomas?

  a. delayed puberty
  b. primary amenorrhea
  c. secondary amenorrhea
  d. galactorrhea

15–5. Which of the following diseases is NOT associated with hyperprolactinemia?

  a. Hand–Schuller–Christian disease
  b. neurofibromatosis
  c. cystic fibrosis
  d. syphilis

15–6. Which of the following is NOT true regarding pituitary tumors?

  a. They occur with a frequency of 5 percent in the general population.
  b. The majority of the lesions are asymptomatic and diagnosed at autopsy.
  c. Lesions have been described that secrete all of the known pituitary trophic hormones.
  d. Prolactinoma is the most common endocrine active tumor.

15–7. Which characteristic best describes the null cell tumor?

  a. It is a rapidly growing, highly invasive tumor.
  b. It usually secretes the peptide adrenocorticotropic hormone (ACTH).
  c. The lesions are usually large and endocrine inactive.
  d. none of the above

15–8. The appropriate evaluation of the patient with a prolactinoma <10 mm in size includes all of the following EXCEPT

  a. serum PRL level
  b. serum TSH level
  c. visual field examination
  d. CT or MRI of the sella turcica

15–9. The most common visual field findings seen with prolactinomas >10 mm in size include

  a. bitemporal hemianopia
  b. normal visual field
  c. unilateral superior temporal hemianopia
  d. superior bitemporal hemianopia

15–10. Bromocriptine therapy has been associated with which of the following side effects?

  a. psychosis
  b. cardiac dysrhythmia
  c. syncope
  d. all of the above

15–11. Which of the following best describes bromocriptine?

  a. It is a dopamine receptor antagonist.
  b. It primarily acts through the D1 receptor.
  c. It inhibits the secretion but not synthesis of PRL.
  d. It will not inhibit PRL secretion from tumors lacking D2 receptors.

15–12. What percentage of patients with Cushing's disease experience irregular menstruation or amenorrhea?

  a. 10 percent
  b. 25 percent

c. 50 percent
d. 75 percent

15–13. Which of the following is NOT associated with growth hormone (GH)-secreting tumors?

a. cardiac, hepatic, and renal enlargement
b. hypotension
c. visual disturbance
d. cardiovascular, cerebrovascular, and respiratory disease

15–14. The stimulation of gonadotropin-secreting pituitary tumors with thyrotropin-releasing hormone (TRH) results in an elevation in which of the following hormones most consistently?

a. follicle-stimulating hormone (FSH)
b. luteinizing hormone (LH)
c. LH-β
d. LH-α

15–15. Which of the following statements best describes craniopharyngioma?

a. The lesions always occur in childhood or adolescence.
b. The tumors are usually less than 5 mm in size.
c. The lesions are slow growing.
d. One half of the lesions are calcified.

15–16. What is the maximal dose of iodinizing radiation the hypothalamus can tolerate?

a. 3000 rads
b. 4500 rads
c. 6000 rads
d. 10,000 rads

15–17. Which of the following disorders can disrupt hypothalamic function?

a. tuberculosis
b. syphilis
c. sarcoidosis
d. all of the above

15–18. The posterior wall of Rathke's pouch gives rise to which level of the pituitary gland?

a. anterior lobe
b. posterior lobe

c. intermediate lobe
d. all of the above

15–19. Melanocyte-stimulating hormone (MSH) has an amino acid structure similar to

a. PRL
b. GH
c. ACTH
d. antidiuretic hormone (ADH)

15–20. Which of the following is associated with pituitary infarction?

a. hemorrhage into the tumor
b. severe headaches
c. rapid loss of vision
d. all of the above

15–21. Large tumors that extend into the hypothalamus have been associated with

a. diabetes insipidus
b. temperature dysregulation
c. satiety regulation
d. all of the above

15–22. What percentage of women experience amenorrhea in association with nonfunctional pituitary tumors?

a. 5 percent
b. 10 percent
c. 15 percent
d. 20 percent

15–23. Which of the following is the most common postoperative complication associated with transsphenoidal hypophysectomy?

a. cerebrospinal fluid leaks
b. bleeding
c. headaches
d. diabetes insipidus

15–24. Carpal tunnel syndrome is associated with the secretion of which pituitary tropic hormone?

a. PRL
b. TSH
c. ACTH
d. GH

15–25. Following the treatment of GH-secreting tumors with radiation, what percentage of patients experience amenorrhea?

    a. 10 percent
    b. 20 percent
    c. 30 percent
    d. 50 percent

15–26. Which of the following pharmaceutical agents has been employed in the medical therapy of acromegaly?

    a. TRH
    b. leuprolide acetate
    c. somatostatin analogs
    d. vasopressin

Chapter 16

ANOVULATION OF CNS ORIGIN: FUNCTIONAL AND MISCELLANEOUS CAUSES

CASE REPORT

The patient is a 24-year-old white female, para 0-0-0-0, who began to have menstrual periods in the 7th grade. Since that time, menstruation has been irregular, and she has been amenorrheic for the last 4 years since discontinuing oral contraceptive agents. It is also noted that in the same year an IUD was placed, she became infected and had to be admitted to the hospital for removal of the IUD and antibiotic therapy. She admits to some nausea and vomiting, and her weight decreased from 120 lb to 101³/₄ lb during this time period. She had episodes of fatigue and palpitations and was thought to have tachycardia in the past. She also had an abnormal glucose tolerance test, and was admitted to the hospital for what was thought to be pancreatitis. There was no remarkable family history. She was married, had graduated from college, and was enrolled in professional school. She smoked and consumed alcohol socially.

Physical examination showed the following: weight, 101³/₄ lb; height, 5'8"; blood pressure, 90/60; pulse, 50; respirations, 20; HEENT, within normal limits; neck, no thyromegaly; heart, regular sinus rhythm; chest, clear; breasts, Tanner stage V; pelvic, normal with a nulliparous cervix, normal-sized uterus, and no adnexal masses.

Laboratory data included a follicle-stimulating hormone (FSH) level of 7.5, luteinizing hormone (LH) 4.5, prolactin (PRL) 2.71 ng/ml, and an estradiol level of 16 pg/ml.

In view of the inappropriate fat/lean mass ratio, anorectoid personality, hypogonadotropic hypogonadism, and inverted LH/FSH ratio, it was felt that she had psychogenic amenorrhea, probably borderline anorexia nervosa, cardiac dysautonomia, and Barlow syndrome. ?

Subsequently, she was evaluated by the department of cardiology; a mid-systolic click was noted. A tilt and Valsalva test confirmed the diagnosis of cardiac dysautonomia. She was also evaluated by the department of clinical nutrition, and it was believed that she probably had anorexia nervosa. Her Minnesota Multiphasic Personality Inventory (MMPI) and clinical history supported that diagnosis, and the clinical picture was one of caloric insufficiency and a moderate degree of emaciation resulting in amenorrhea. Subsequently, she was evaluated further by the cardiology department and was noted to have swelling of her legs and pitting edema. At that time, her resting heart rate was 65 beats/min, and she had an unusually marked degree of sinus arrhythmia which far exceeded that generally seen in the adult population. The sinus mechanism was capable of accelerating to rates of 90 beats/min on abrupt change in position; however, her response was very inappropriate in that after increasing her heart rate 30 percent, on assuming the upright posture, she developed an inappropriate heart rate that was only 7 percent greater than her recumbent heart rate. This accounted for her tendency to feel weak upon changing position. She also had an abnormal blood pressure regulation mechanism, in that rather than having a slight increase in blood pressure, which would have been appropriate, she maintained a resting pressure of 90/60, which changed to 85/65 on standing. Doppler flow studies of the radial artery showed an unusually marked decrease in the amplitude of the signal during the standing position, indicative of a patient with a marked predominance of vagal tone. During the Valsalva maneuver, she showed no tachycardia throughout the straining position, and her heart rate increased only mildly after releasing the intrathoracic pressure. In spite of the fact that her blood pressure changed only from 90/60 to 100/60 during the post-strain phase, she developed inappropriate prolonged bradycardia in the post-strain phase. This kind of test with the absence of tachycardia during the strain is seen in patients with marked vagal tone.

In view of the fact that patients with this type of autonomic response complain of easy fatigability and progressive weakness, particularly when they exert themselves, small-dose phenobarbital therapy was initiated to reduce the vagal tone centrally by acting on the limbic system and midbrain.

After an absence of 2 years, during which time the patient rejected her diagnosis, she returned seeking pregnancy. She was begun on Pergonal therapy at 150 mIU/day. After receiving five doses of Pergonal, her estradiol level had increased to 127 pg/ml. She was treated for 2 more days with 150 mIU, after which her estrogen level had increased to 211 ng/ml. She was treated for an additional 2 days with 150 IU. At that juncture, her estradiol level had reached 1,395 pg/ml, and she had moderate cervical mucus and adequate spinnbarkeit. She was given 10,000 units of human chorionic gonadotropin (hCG) and failed to conceive in the primary treatment cycle. Subsequently, she was again treated for 5 days with 150 IU of Pergonal, and her estrogen level was 114 ng/ml. She was treated for 2 more days at the same dose, and her level had increased to 560 pg/ml. She had adequate cervical mucus, was given 1 further day of therapy, and received 10,000 units of hCG. Subsequently, she was treated with two 2,000-unit boosters of hCG spaced

at 5-day intervals, but failed to conceive. Following this cycle, therapy was stopped for 3 months, during which time she was cycled on 1.25 mg of Premarin on days 1 to 25 and 10 mg of Provera on days 16 to 25. Unfortunately, during this time period, she lost an additional 5 lb. Subsequently, she was restarted on Pergonal therapy at 225 IU and had an estradiol level of 56 pg/ml after 5 days of therapy. She was treated with 4 more days of therapy, at which time her estradiol level was 371 pg/ml. The patient failed to come in for evaluation of her estradiol level but wished to continue therapy. She was treated for 1 further day, and her estradiol level was determined to be 1,178 pg/ml. Cervical mucus was thin, and she was given 10,000 units of hCG. She was treated in this cycle with progesterone suppositories at 25 mg/day during the luteal phase. Unfortunately, conception failed to occur. Subsequently, she was restarted on Pergonal, was treated with 150 units/day for 4 days, and her estradiol level was 132 pg/ml. She was treated for an additional 2 days and presented with an estradiol level of 400 pg/ml. A sonar scan at that time did not demonstrate the presence of maturing follicles. The Pergonal dose was increased to 225 units/day for 3 days, and she was given 10,000 units of hCG. She failed to ovulate in this cycle and demonstrated a progesterone level of 1.1 ng/ml on cycle day 22. She was treated with an additional Pergonal cycle at 225 IU/day, and after 5 days her estradiol level was 248 pg/ml. She was given 2 more days of therapy; her estradiol level was 196 pg/ml at that juncture. The dose was increased to 2 amps/day; following 5 further days of therapy, her estradiol level had increased to 1,875 pg/ml, and she had two mature follicles present on the right ovary. Ovulation was induced with 10,000 units of hCG on cycle day 16, and she was treated with 25 mg of progesterone vaginal suppositories during the luteal phase. She was able to conceive in this cycle. Sonar scan showed an intrauterine pregnancy, but fetal activity could not be seen. She was rescanned in 2 weeks, at which time a twin gestation at 10 weeks and 4 days was identified. She was continued on progesterone therapy and was rescanned 2 weeks later, at which time a quadruplet gestation was identified with positive fetal heartbeats (Fig 16–1). The patient was hospitalized at 6 months' gestation, where she remained on bedrest throughout the remainder of the pregnancy. It was observed that she would sit in her room and repeatedly watch the videotape of the

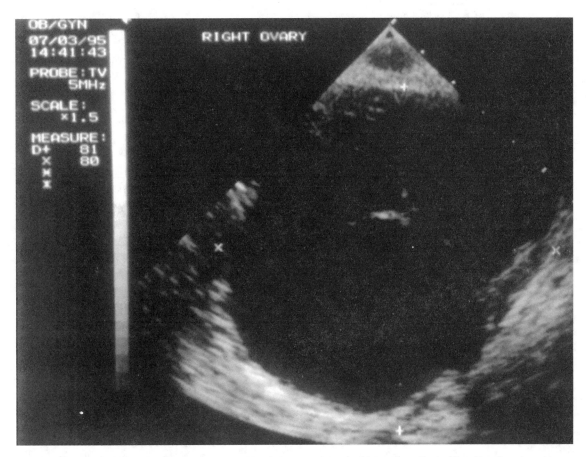

Figure 16–1. Quadruplet gestation resulting from gonadotropin therapy in patient with eating disorder.

sonar of the quadruplets. Subsequently, she delivered by cesarean section a term set of quadruplets at 38 weeks. The babies were discharged without incident after a brief stay in the nursery.

SUMMARY AND CONCLUSIONS

The psychogenic amenorrheas usually result from one of three things: stress, an altered body weight, and increased physical activity, or a combination of all three. Deviation from ideal body weight by about 15 percent or more produces menstrual dysfunction. In fact, correction of body weight can result in pregnancy rates as high as 68 percent with no other management. Anorexia nervosa was first described by Richard Morton in 1869. He depicted a 17-year-old girl with nervous consumption as follows: "I do not remember that I did ever in all my practice see one that was conversant with the living, so much wasted with the greatest degree of consumption (like a skeleton, only clad with skin), yet there was no fever but on the contrary coldness

of the whole body . . ." This disorder occurs in teenagers who lose more than 25 percent of their body weight. Menstrual dysfunction usually occurs prior to weight loss, and if the individual is able to regain weight, often they will still have disordered menstruation. The weight loss is accompanied by a fear of obesity, body image disturbance, or refusal to gain weight, and often depression. Physical findings include hypotension, hypothermia, bradycardia, cachexia, bradypenia, parotid enlargement, peripheral edema (secondary to hyperalbuminemia), increased body hair, and hyperkeratinemia. These women develop a prepubertal gonadotropin pattern with an inverted FSH/LH pattern, an increased response to gonadotropin-releasing hormone (GnRH), normal or increased cortisol levels, increased levels of reverse triiodothyronine (T_3), decreased dehydroepiandrosterone (DHEA) and dehydroepiandrosterone sulfate (DHEAS) levels, decreased levels of estrogen production, and altered antidiuretic hormone secretion.

As demonstrated by this case, patients who have hypothalamic dysfunction are very responsive to therapy with gonadotropins. Pregnancy rates as high as 30 percent per cycle have been reported, and it should be noted that high-order multiples occur as frequently in women with low body weight as with the "PCO" (polycystic ovary)-like patient.

BIBLIOGRAPHY

Costello RT. Subclinical adenoma of the pituitary gland. *Am J Pathol.* 12:205, 1936

Kovacs K, Horvath E. Pathology of pituitary tumors. *Endocrinol Metab Clin N Am.* 16:529, 1987

Kwekkeboon DJ, de Jong FH, Lamberts SWJ. Gonadotropin release by clinically nonfunctioning and gonadotroph pituitary adenomas in vivo and in vitro: relation to sex and effects of thyrotropin-releasing hormone, gonadotropin-releasing hormone, and bromocriptine. *J Clin Endocrinol Metab.* 68:1128, 1989

Molitch ME. Pathologic hyperprolactinemia. *Endocrinol Metab Clin N Am.* 21:877, 1991

Molitch ME, Elton RL, Blackwell RE, et al. Bromocriptine as primary therapy for prolactin-secreting macroadenomas: results of a prospective multicenter study. *J Clin Endocrinol Metab.* 60:698, 1985

QUESTIONS

16–1. Ovulation can be disrupted by

    a. increased level of stress
    b. decrease in body weight
    c. increase in exercise
    d. all of the above

16–2. Amenorrheic athletes compared to sedentary women have which of the following hormone changes?

    a. decreased total thyroxine levels
    b. decreased free thyroxine levels
    c. increased free T_3 levels
    d. none of the above

16–3. Which of the following changes in thyroid dynamics is found in athletic women?

    a. thyroid-stimulating hormone (TSH) response to thyrotropin-releasing factor (TRF) is blunted
    b. decrease in thyroxine-binding globulin (TBG) level
    c. increase in sex hormone-binding globulin (SHBG) level
    d. decrease in TSH level

16–4. Which of the following is an appropriate initial laboratory test for the evaluation of ovulatory disorders?

    a. LH/FSH
    b. PRL
    c. TSH
    d. all of the above

16–5. Which of the following does not correlate with hypothalamic amenorrhea?

    a. decreased LH/FSH levels
    b. estradiol levels less than 40 pg/ml
    c. an endometrium of 1-cm thickness
    d. a decreased SHBG

16–6. The standard dose of GnRH used to carry out a pituitary challenge test is

    a. 100 µg IV
    b. 200 µg IV
    c. 400 µg IV
    d. 500 µg IV

16–7. Which of the following hormones is unaffected by stress?

    a. PRL
    b. oxytocin
    c. vasopressin
    d. none of the above

16–8. Which of the following hormones does NOT inhibit GnRH/LH secretion?

    a. corticotropin-releasing hormone (CRH)
    b. thyrotropin-releasing hormone (TRH)
    c. oxytocin
    d. none of the above

16–9. During the first 3 years of amenorrhea, bone density would be expected to decrease

    a. 1 percent
    b. 5 percent
    c. 7 to 10 percent
    d. 15 percent

16–10. Which of the following ovulation induction profiles is generally NOT effective in the patient with hypothalamic amenorrhea?

   a. low-dose clomiphene, 25 mg/day for 5 days

   b. human menopausal gonadotropin (hMG), 150 IU/day

   c. native GnRH, 5 mg/90 min

   d. clomiphene citrate, 100 mg/day for 5 days

16–11. The mortality associated with anorexia is

   a. 1 percent

   b. 5 percent

   c. 9 percent

   d. 15 percent

16–12. Which of the following is NOT associated with the diagnostic criteria for anorexia nervosa?

   a. fear of obesity

   b. body image disturbance

   c. loss of 25 percent of body weight

   d. voluntary attempt to gain weight

16–13. Which of the following is NOT a physical finding associated with anorexia nervosa?

   a. hypotension

   b. hypothermia

   c. tachycardia

   d. hyperkeratinemia

16–14. Which of the following laboratory studies is found in the patient with anorexia nervosa?

   a. inverted FSH/LH ratio

   b. decreased cortisol level

   c. increased DHEA level

   d. decreased reverse T_3 level

16–15. According to the Frisch nomogram, what percentage of body fat is necessary for normal menstruation?

   a. 5 percent

   b. 10 percent

   c. 15 percent

   d. 22 percent

16–16. The association of hypoestrogenism and psychic factors was described in 1943 by

   a. Klinefelter

   b. Pincus and Rock

   c. Corner

   d. Shally

16–17. Which of the following is derived from the metabolism pro-opiomelantocortin?

   a. alpha melanocyte-stimulating hormone (α-MSH)

   b. adrenocorticotropic hormone (ACTH)

   c. β-endorphin

   d. all of the above

16–18. Which physiologist proposed the general adaption syndrome?

   a. Hans Selye

   b. Claude Bernard

   c. Charles Sherrington

   d. William Beaumont

16–19. The minimum dose of estrogen replacement that conserves bone density in a population two standard deviations from the mean is

   a. 0.3 mg conjugated estrogen

   b. 0.625 mg conjugated estrogen

   c. 0.9 mg conjugated estrogen

   d. 1 mg micronized estradiol

16–20. Which of the following is true regarding eating disorders?

   a. Patients tend to be Caucasian.

   b. Patients tend to be from the upper to middle class.

   c. Bulimic behavior occurs in 18 percent of high school and college students.

   d. all of the above

16–21. According to the Diagnostic and Statistical Manual, 4th edition (DSM-IV), bulimia nervosa occurs in what percentage of the female population?

   a. 1 to 2 percent

   b. 5 percent

   c. 10 percent

   d. 15 percent

16–22. What activity results in the highest incidence of reproductive dysfunction?

 a. cycling
 b. swimming
 c. weight lifting
 d. long-distance running

16–23. Which of the following menstrual abnormalities has been described in runners?

 a. luteal-phase defect
 b. loss of mid-cycle LH surge
 c. prolonged menstrual cycle
 d. all of the above

16–24. Which of the following is characteristic of pseudocyesis?

 a. morning sickness
 b. amenorrhea
 c. increased abdominal girth
 d. all of the above

16–25. Which of the following hormonal abnormalities has been observed in pseudocyesis?

 a. decrease in PRL level
 b. increase in LH level
 c. increase in FSH level
 d. decrease in antidiuretic hormone (ADH) level

16–26. Kallmann syndrome is inherited as a(an)

 a. autosomal recessive pattern
 b. autosomal dominant pattern
 c. X-linked pattern
 d. multifactor

17

THYROID DYSFUNCTION AND OVULATORY DISORDERS

CASE REPORT

The patient is a 19-year-old white female, para 0-0-0-0, who underwent menarche at 11 years of age. She presents with a history of irregular menstrual cycles over the past 12 months, increased weight gain, and bilateral pelvic pain. The pain is central, intermittent, and cramping. There has been no change in bowel function. There has also been no change in urinary function, although bladder capacity appears to be slightly diminished. The patient denies any intake of medication, does not use recreational drugs, smoke, or drink alcohol. Physical examination shows a well-nourished, 180-lb, 5'4^1/$_2$", white female. No thyromegaly is demonstrated, nor is galactorrhea. Ferriman–Gallwey score is 1. Pelvic examination is normal with the exception of enlarged cystic adnexa.

A urine pregnancy test is negative. Transvaginal sonography demonstrates enlarged cystic adnexa, 8 to 10 cm (Fig 17–1). Her luteinizing hormone (LH) was 7 mIU/ml, follicle-stimulating hormone (FSH) 5 mIU/ml, prolactin (PRL) 10 ng/ml, and thyroid-stimulating hormone (TSH) 14 mIU/ml.

The patient is diagnosed as having compensated hypothyroidism and functional ovarian cysts. She was started simultaneously on levothyroxine sodium (Synthroid) 100 mg/day and norethindrone acetate (Norlutate) 15 mg/day for 2 weeks. Repeat sonography carried out at the end of 2 weeks shows resolution of the ovarian cyst and normal-sized ovaries. A TSH level was found to be 4 mIU/ml. Following discontinuation of Norlutate therapy, the patient resumed monthly menstruation on Synthroid replacement therapy.

SUMMARY AND CONCLUSIONS

Ovarian cyst formation, regardless of the etiology, should be managed conservatively. There is little place for surgery, even of an endoscopic variety, in the management of these problems. The patient with such a presentation should be evaluated for pregnancy and either be treated expectantly with management of her pain symptoms or undergo ovarian suppression with high-dose progestogen therapy. It should be noted that the use of low-dose oral contraceptive therapy has not been shown to be any more efficient than expectant management in the treatment of ovarian cysts. Further, the currently used low-dose oral contraceptive agents do not block folliculogenesis, only ovulation. In fact, one finds an inverse relationship between the amount of ethinyl estradiol contained in a birth control pill and 17β-estradiol production.

Further, this case demonstrates that subtle increases in TSH production, which is diagnostic for compensated hypothyroidism, often result in ovulatory dysfunction. The high-sensitivity TSH determination has largely replaced other thyroid function studies in the diagnosis of this disorder.

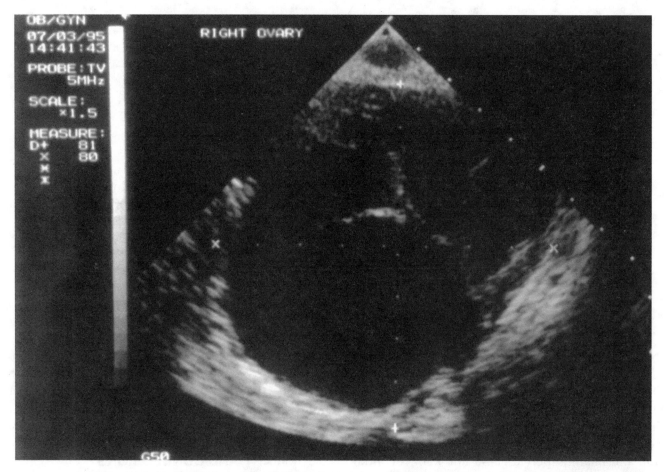

Figure 17–1. Transvaginal sonogram of multicystic ovary in a patient with compensated hypothyroidism.

BIBLIOGRAPHY

Erfurth EM, Ericsson UB. The role of estrogen in the TSH and prolactin responses to thyrotropin-releasing hormone in postmenopausal as compared to premenopausal women. *Horm Metab Res.* 24(11):528, 1992

Girdler SS, Pedersen CA, Light KC. Thyroid axis function during the menstrual cycle in women with premenstrual syndrome. *Psychoneuroendocrinology.* 20(4):395, 1995

Sarne DH, Degroot LJ. Hypothalamic and neuroendocrine regulation of thyroid hormone. In: DeGroot LJ, ed. *Endocrinology,* 2nd ed. Philadelphia, PA, W. B. Saunders, 1989: 574–589

Sawin CT, Hershman JM, Boyd AE III, et al. The relationship of change in serum estradiol and progesterone during the menstrual cycle to the thyrotropin and prolactin responses to thyrotropin-releasing hormone. *J Clin Endocrinol Metab.* 47:1296, 1978

Utiger RD. Hypothyroidism. In: DeGroot LJ, ed. *Endocrinology,* 2nd ed. Philadelphia, PA, W. B. Saunders, 1989: 702–721

QUESTIONS

17–1. Which of the following is true regarding the embryology of the thyroid gland?

    a. It is the first endocrine gland to appear embryologically.

    b. It begins formation at 14 days after fertilization.

    c. A pyramidal lobe is present in 50 percent of patients.

    d. all of the above

17–2. The gene for thyroglobulin has been mapped to chromosome

    a. 2

    b. 8

    c. 16

    d. 22

17–3. Thyroid hormones circulate bound to

    a. thyroxine-binding globulin (TBG)
    b. thyroxine-binding prealbumin
    c. albumin
    d. all of the above

17–4. Which of the following results in a decrease in peripheral triiodothyronine (T_3) production?

    a. starvation
    b. diabetes mellitus
    c. somatostatin therapy
    d. all of the above

17–5. Which of the following agents reduces T_3 conversion?

    a. propylthiouracil ✓
    b. prazosine
    c. amiodarone
    d. all of the above

17–6. Which of the following is the most useful test in determining the state of hypothyroidism?

    a. high-sensitivity TSH
    b. serum T_3
    c. serum thyroxine (T_4)
    d. T_3 uptake

17–7. TSH secretion is inhibited by

    a. norepinephrine
    b. arginine vasopressin
    c. thinelferin
    d. somatostatin

17–8. Which of the following is the rate-limiting step in TSH production?

    a. the synthesis of the α-subunit
    b. the synthesis of the β-subunit
    c. the coupling of α- and β-subunits
    d. none of the above

17–9. The response of TSH to thyrotropin-releasing factor (TRF) stimulation is blunted by

    a. somatostatin
    b. glucocorticoids
    c. dopamine agonists
    d. all of the above

17–10. In the state of hypothyroidism

    a. gonadotropins are unchanged
    b. gonadotropins are decreased
    c. gonadotropins are elevated
    d. only FSH is elevated

17–11. Glucocorticoid therapy in large doses affects thyroid dynamics by

    a. decreasing TSH secretion
    b. decreasing the peripheral conversion of T_4 to T_3
    c. reducing TBG levels
    d. all of the above

17–12. The incidence of hypothyroidism in women is

    a. 40 percent
    b. 20 percent
    c. 10 percent
    d. 5 percent

17–13. Which of the following is NOT a cause of hypothyroidism?

    a. autoimmune thyroiditis
    b. thyroid dysgenesis
    c. infiltrative thyroid disease
    d. none of the above

17–14. Postpartum hypothyroidism occurs in what percentage of women?

    a. 40 percent
    b. 25 percent
    c. 10 percent
    d. 3 percent

17–15. Which of the following forms of hypothyroidism occurs in the older patient?

    a. Graves' disease
    b. Hashimoto's thyroiditis
    c. toxic nodular goiter
    d. silent thyroiditis

17–16. Pretibial myxedema occurs in what percentage of patients with Graves' disease?

    a. 25 percent
    b. 15 percent
    c. 10 percent
    d. 4 percent

17–17. Primary hypothyroidism is associated with

  a. delayed puberty
  b. precocious puberty
  c. ovarian cysts
  d. all of the above

17–18. Hyperthyroidism is associated with

  a. delayed puberty
  b. precocious puberty
  c. amenorrhea
  d. all of the above

17–19. Which of the following is true regarding iodide transport and assimilation?

  a. Iodide is actively transported from serum by a membrane-associated pump.
  b. Concentrations of the follicle cell are fivefold that of serum.
  c. TSH does not stimulate this gradient.
  d. Iodide remains free in the follicular cell for days before being assimilated.

17–20. Which of the following is true regarding iodide metabolism?

  a. Iodide must be reduced prior to incorporation into thyroglobulin.
  b. Thyroglobulin has a molecular weight of about 200,000.
  c. Thyroid peroxidase, a membrane-bound enzyme, catalyzes the electron transfer from iodide.
  d. Thyroglobulin normally contains four iodothyronine sites per molecule.

17–21. Which of the following is true regarding thyroglobulin?

  a. It contains units of monoiodothyronine.
  b. It contains units of diiodothyronine.
  c. Subunits are coupled by diethinyl ether linkages to form T_4 and T_3.
  d. all of the above

17–22. Which of the following binding proteins has the greatest affinity for thyroxine?

  a. TBG
  b. thyroxine-binding prealbumin
  c. albumin
  d. sex hormone-binding globulin

17–23. Which of the following hormones has the lowest daily production rate?

  a. T_4
  b. T_3
  c. monoiodothyronine (MIT)
  d. reverse T_3

17–24. Which of the following organ systems receives the largest distribution of T_4?

  a. liver and kidney
  b. muscle, brain, and skin
  c. plasma
  d. bone

17–25. Thyroid hormones

  a. stimulate gluconeogenesis
  b. stimulate lipogenesis
  c. regulate thermogenesis
  d. all of the above

17–26. Thyroid hormones act on all of these cellular sites EXCEPT the

  a. cell membrane
  b. mitochondria
  c. nucleus
  d. Golgi apparatus

17–27. Which of the following are muscle symptoms associated with hypothyroidism?

  a. pain and cramps
  b. proximal weakness
  c. slow reflexes
  d. all of the above

Chapter 18

DISORDERS OF THE ADRENAL CORTEX

CASE REPORT

A 5-year-old girl was referred to Children's Medical Center for evaluation of clitoral enlargement. The child was born following an uncomplicated pregnancy and delivery. At birth, the child was noted to have a large clitoris but was not evaluated further. The child had no other medical complaints and denied previous surgery.

The physical examination revealed a child who appeared tall for her age (height, 3'2"; weight, 61 lb, 6 oz). There was no breast development and no axillary hair.

Her pelvic exam revealed the presence of pubic hair and an enlarged clitoris (Fig 18–1). A single perineal opening was detected below the clitoris.

An abdominal ultrasound revealed the presence of small ovaries and a uterus. A chromosome analysis was obtained and revealed a 46,XX karyotype. Serum testosterone was 1.2 ng/ml, androstenedione was 4.2 ng/ml, and 17-OH progesterone was 92 ng/ml. Based on these tests results, the diagnosis of congenital 21-hydroxylase deficiency, simple virilizing type, was made. The child was begun on therapy with hydrocortisone. A decision was made to proceed with a clitoral reduction and vulvoplasty (Fig 18–2).

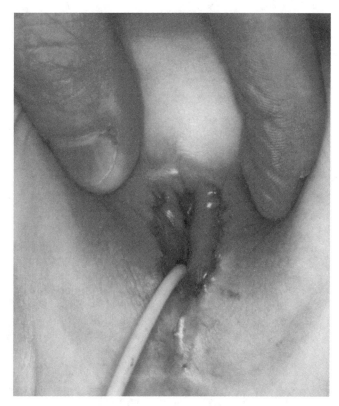

Figure 18–1. Virilized external genitalia of a 5-year-old female with 21-hydroxylase deficiency. *(Courtesy of Dr. Karen D. Bradshaw, University of Texas Southwestern Medical Center at Dallas, Dallas, TX.)*

Figure 18–2. Immediate postoperative repair of clitoral reduction and vulvoplasty. *(Courtesy of Dr. Karen D. Bradshaw, University of Texas Southwestern Medical Center at Dallas, Dallas, TX.)*

Table 18–1. Phenotype in 21-Hydroxylase Deficiency

Characteristic	Salt wasting	Simple virilizing	Nonclassic form
Age at diagnosis	Infancy	Infancy (females) or childhood (males)	Childhood or adulthood
Aldosterone	Low	Normal	Normal
Virilization	Severe to moderate	Moderate to severe	None to mild
Mutation	Severe	Moderate (severe + moderate)	Mild (mild + moderate, mild + severe)

Adapted from Speiser PW. Congenital adrenal hyperplasia. In: Becker KL, ed. *Endocrinology and Metabolism.* J. B. Lippincott, Philadelphia, PA, 1995: 687–693.

Vaginoplasty to open the urogenital sinus will be done in the late teenage years when the patient can successfully work with vaginal dilators.

SUMMARY AND CONCLUSIONS

Deficiency of P_{450C21} accounts for the majority of cases of congenital sexual ambiguity, but a smaller number of adults with androgen excess. The phenotypes of 21-hydroxylase are depicted in Table 18–1. Of the various phenotypes for 21-hydroxylase deficiency, the salt wasting form accounts for about 75 percent of the cases. Simple virilizing forms account for 25 percent of cases. Usually, the diagnosis is made at birth, but, if unrecognized, the subject will continue to show signs of progressive virilization and accelerated height. In most cases, aldosterone synthesis is near normal and prevents salt wasting. A number of mutations of the 21-hydroxylase gene have been described. Treatment includes hydrocortisone to suppress adrenal androgen secretion, and when this is controlled one can proceed with clitoral reduction and vaginoplasty.

BIBLIOGRAPHY

Aisenberg JE, Speiser PW. The genetics of 21-hydroxylase deficiency. *Endocrinologist.* 4:92, 1994

New MI, White PC, Pang S, Dupont B, Speiser PW. The adrenal hyperplasias. In: Scriver CR, Beaudet AL, Sly WS, Valle D, eds. *The Metabolic Basis of Inherited Disease,* 6th ed. New York, McGraw-Hill, 1989:380–388.

Speiser PW, Dupont J, Zhu D, et al. Disease expression and molecular genotype in congenital adrenal hyperplasia due to 21-hydroxylase deficiency. *J Clin Invest.* 90:584, 1992

White PC, New MI. Genetic basis of endocrine disease 2: congenital adrenal hyperplasia due to 21-hydroxylase deficiency. *J Clin Endocrinol Metab.* 74:6, 1992

White PC, New MI, Dupont B. Structure of the human steroid 21-hydroxylase genes. *Proc Natl Acad Sci USA.* 83:5111, 1986

QUESTIONS

18–1. Which of the following is NOT a P_{450} enzyme found in the adrenal cortex?

   a. cholesterol side-chain cleavage
   b. 3β-hydroxysteroid dehydrogenase
   c. 17α-hydroxylase
   d. 21-hydroxylase

18–2. Which of the following is true regarding 21-hydroxylase?

   a. Activity is present in granulosa cells.
   b. The gene is located on chromosome 4.
   c. A pseudogene is located on the long arm of chromosome 4.
   d. none of the above

18–3. Which of the following enzyme activities are located in the zona glomerulosa?

   a. 18-hydroxylase
   b. 17α-hydroxylase
   c. 17,20-lyase
   d. all of the above

18–4. Following chronic stress such as occurs in burn patients, which of the following exists?

   a. cortisol increases, dehydroepiandrosterone sulfate (DHEAS) increases
   b. cortisol decreases, DHEAS increases
   c. cortisol decreases, DHEAS decreases
   d. cortisol increases, DHEAS decreases

18–5. What is the dose of adrenocorticotropic hormone (ACTH) used in an ACTH stimulation test?

   a. 100 mg
   b. 250 mg
   c. 100 µg
   d. 250 µg

18–6. Desoxycorticosterone (DOC) is secreted primarily by which zone of the adrenal cortex?

   a. zona glomerulosa
   b. zona fasciculata
   c. zona reticularis
   d. medulla

18–7. In postmenopausal women, which of the following is true?

   a. DHEA levels are higher than those in men.
   b. DHEAS levels are lower than those in men.
   c. DHEA levels are lower than those in men.
   d. DHEAS levels are higher than those in men.

18–8. Glucocorticoids induce

   a. decreased hepatic glycogen deposition
   b. hypoglycemia
   c. positive protein balance
   d. negative calcium balance

18–9. Which of the following glucocorticoids is the most potent?

   a. prednisone
   b. hydrocortisone
   c. dexamethasone
   d. prednisolone

18–10. Which of the following is characteristic of ectopic ACTH production?

   a. It accounts for approximately 10 percent of Cushing syndrome.
   b. It occurs most commonly in men.
   c. The oat cell tumor is the primary source.
   d. all of the above

18–11. Which of the following tests results essentially rules out Cushing syndrome?

   a. 8 AM cortisol, 8 µg/dl
   b. 8 AM cortisol, 3 µg/dl, after overnight dexamethasone 1 mg suppression
   c. 24-hour urinary free cortisol of 90 µg
   d. all of the above

18–12. Which of the following is true for an ectopic ACTH source?

   a. inferior petrosal sinus (IPS)/peripheral gradient ≥2
   b. corticotropin-releasing hormone (CRH)-stimulated ACTH release is 100 percent above basal values
   c. best diagnosed by CT scan
   d. none of the above

18–13. Which of the following is true concerning Nelson syndrome?

   a. high ACTH levels
   b. hyperpigmentation
   c. visual loss
   d. all of the above

18–14. The metyrapone test

   a. inhibits 17α-hydroxylase activity
   b. is used to diagnose Cushing syndrome
   c. increases endogenous ACTH levels
   d. all of the above

18–15. In an infant with 3β-hydroxysteroid dehydrogenase deficiency, which of the following is true?

   a. a rare cause of congenital adrenal hyperplasia
   b. low levels of DHEA
   c. low levels of DHEAS
   d. high basal levels of 17-hydroxyprogesterone

18–16. The characteristics of simple virilizing 21-hydroxylase activity include

   a. age at diagnosis in females is childhood
   b. low aldosterone levels
   c. moderate to severe virilization
   d. mild to moderate mutation

18–17. Simple virilizing accounts for what percentage of all virilizing 21-hydroxylase deficiency cases?

   a. 10 percent
   b. 25 percent
   c. 50 percent
   d. 75 percent

18–18. Which of the following is a 21 carbon steroid?

    a. aldosterone
    b. DOC
    c. pregnenolone
    d. all of the above

18–19. Which of the following is a mineralocorticoid?

    a. DOC
    b. corticosterone
    c. aldosterone
    d. all of the above

18–20. CRH contains how many peptides?

    a. 10
    b. 21
    c. 39
    d. 41

18–21. β-Endorphin is the direct metabolic product of which of the following hormones?

    a. ACTH
    b. pro-opiomelanocortin (POMC)
    c. α-endorphin
    d. β-lipotropin

18–22. Which of the following hormones acts synergistically to release CRH, which leads to ACTH and cortisol formation?

    a. serotonin
    b. β-lipotropin
    c. growth hormone
    d. none of the above

18–23. Which of the following is NOT true regarding cortisol?

    a. half-life of 2 hours
    b. production rate of 10 mg/day
    c. metabolized to tetrahydrocortisone
    d. free cortisol is 10 percent

18–24. All of the following are true regarding protein binding of cortisol EXCEPT

    a. 1 percent free
    b. 30 percent bound to albumin
    c. 60 percent bound to cortisol-binding globulin (CBG)
    d. all of the above

18–25. Increased free cortisol is found in

    a. oral contraceptive treatment
    b. acromegaly
    c. pregnancy
    d. all of the above

18–26. Which of the following increases aldosterone secretion?

    a. CRH
    b. angiotensin
    c. hyperkalemia
    d. all of the above

18–27. What percentage of circulating DHEAS is produced by the adrenal cortex?

    a. 5 percent
    b. 50 percent
    c. 90 percent
    d. 98 percent

Chapter 19

OVARIAN DYSFUNCTION AND ANOVULATION

CASE REPORT

The patient is a 25-year-old white female, para 0-0-0-0, with a history of menarche at 12 years of age. She gives a lifelong history of irregular menstruation and has cycle lengths that range from 26 to 45 days. She complains of increasing hirsutism and weight gain. Her sister has a similar problem and has been told she has polycystic ovary syndrome (PCOS).

Physical examination shows a 5'3", 190-lb white female, with a Ferriman–Gallwey score of 10. The patient is found to have dark hairs on the chin, upper lip, and around the areola, and has a male escutcheon. Her luteinizing hormone (LH) level is 10 mIU/ml and follicle-stimulating hormone (FSH) level is 3 mIU/ml; thyroid-stimulating hormone (TSH), dehydroepiandrosterone sulfate (DHEAS), and 17-hydroxyprogesterone (17-OHP) are normal. Total testosterone is 90 ng/dl, free testosterone is 1.25 ng/dl, and sex hormone-binding globulin (SHBG) is 14 µ/L. The patient has a negative urinary pregnancy test, is given progesterone in oil, and withdraws with bleeding.

She is treated with 150 mg of clomiphene citrate (Serophene) on days 2 to 6, as she has been treated with up to 100 mg for 3 days in the past. She failed to ovulate on triple Serophene, was subsequently treated with 150 mg of Serophene, underwent sonography on cycle day 16, had a 1.8- and 2.2-cm follicle, and was given 10,000 units of human chorionic gonadotropin (hCG). This course of therapy was repeated for three cycles with follicles ranging from 1.8 to 1.9 cm. Hysterosalpingogram was carried out, which was normal; postcoital test timed to the hCG injection was also normal.

The patient underwent a diagnostic laparoscopy and was found to have stage I endometriosis, which was treated by excision and confirmation of polycystic ovaries (Fig 19–1). Subsequently, the patient postponed gonadotropin therapy, choosing to reduce her body weight. On her first treatment cycle with Fertinex (urofollitropin), she developed moderate hyperstimulation syndrome with 5- to 6-cm ovaries and rested from therapy for two cycles. She developed a spontaneous pregnancy, with her last menstrual period being May 26. Sonar scan done on July 11 showed a 0.4-cm gestational sac with a 1-cm endometrium. Subsequent sonar scan done on July 15 showed a twin gestation with markedly dissimilar sacs; no crown–rump lengths were visible. This was confirmed on August 12, and the patient underwent a suction dilation and curettage (D&C) procedure.

SUMMARY AND CONCLUSIONS

The diagnosis of PCOS is controversial. In Europe, sonography is often used to make the diagnosis, whereas in the continental United States, the diagnosis is usually rendered by laboratory evaluation. The much-touted elevated LH/FSH ratio is found

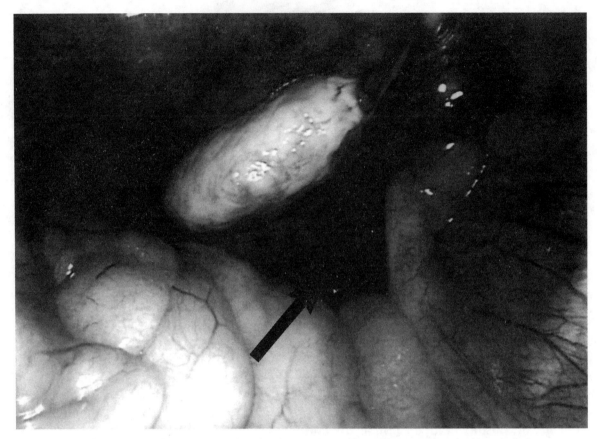

Figure 19–1. Laparoscopic image of polycystic ovary in a patient with concomitant endometriosis (see arrow).

only 40 percent of the time, and often these patients will have an upper limit of normal total testosterone. However, the free testosterone level is usually elevated, and the SHBG is always decreased.

Historically, ovarian wedge resection produced ovulation greater than 70 percent of the time; however, this surgical procedure was associated with the formation of significant ovarian adhesions. Following the introduction of clomiphene citrate, it was demonstrated that the majority of patients respond to this therapy in dose ranges of 50 mg to 250 mg per day. As demonstrated by this patient, many individuals treated with clomiphene citrate will develop adequate follicle size, yet fail to generate an LH surge. The administration of 10,000 units of hCG will often correct this problem. This patient's pregnancy outcome also points to another unfortunate clinical finding in patients with PCOS, that is, an increased miscarriage rate regardless of the type of medications used to induce ovulation.

BIBLIOGRAPHY

Barnes RB, Lobo RA. Central opioid activity in polycystic ovary syndrome (PCO) with and without dopaminergic modulation. *J Clin Endocrinol Metab.* 61:779, 1985

Conway GS, Agrawal R, Betteridge DJ, Jacobs HS. Risk factors for coronary artery disease in lean and obese women with the polycystic ovary syndrome. *Clin Endocrinol.* 37:119, 1992

Erickson GF, Hsueh AJW, Quigley ME, et al. Functional studies of aromatase activity in human granulosa cells from normal and polycystic ovaries. *J Clin Endocrinol Metab.* 49:514, 1983

Kazer RR, Kessel B, Yen SSC. Circulating luteinizing hormone pulse frequency in women with polycystic ovary syndrome. *J Clin Endocrinol Metab.* 65:233, 1987

Rivier C, Rivier J, Vale W. Stress induced inhibition of reproductive functions: role of endogenous corticotropin-releasing factor. *Science.* 231:607, 1986

QUESTIONS

19–1. The elevated LH/FSH ratio frequently seen in patients with PCOS occurs what percentage of the time?

   a. 10 percent
   b. 20 percent
   c. 30 percent
   d. 40 percent

19–2. Which statement best describes the functional dynamics of LH/FSH secretion in PCOS?

   a. Frequent blood sampling reveals exaggerated pulses of LH in association with low normal levels of FSH.
   b. Estradiol infusion exerts a negative inhibition on both LH and FSH secretion.
   c. The administration of clomiphene citrate elicits an amplified LH rise when compared with controls.
   d. PCOS patients possess a normal response to gonadotropin-releasing hormone (GnRH) administration.

19–3. In arcuate nucleus lesioned monkeys, the infusion of GnRH produces which of the following dynamics?

   a. Continuous infusion of GnRH produces downregulation of gonadotropins.
   b. Increasing GnRH amplitude while maintaining pulse frequency reduces FSH levels but has little effect on LH.
   c. Increasing the GnRH pulse interval while maintaining the dose results in a reduction of LH levels.
   d. all of the above

19–4. Which of the following statements is true regarding endogenous opioids in PCOS?

   a. Administration of naloxone increases LH secretion.
   b. Infusion of β-endorphins suppresses elevated LH levels.
   c. β-Endorphins increase hypothalamic dopamine turnover.
   d. PCOS patients have been found to have an elevated peripheral level of β-endorphin.

19–5. Administration of bromocriptine or dopamine agonists causes what effect on the patient with PCOS?

   a. decreases prolactin (PRL) and increases integrated LH secretion
   b. decreases PRL and increases adrenocorticotropic hormone (ACTH) secretion
   c. increases PRL and decreases ACTH secretion
   d. decreases PRL and integrated LH secretion

19–6. Which of the following statements is true with regard to the polycystic ovary?

   a. Follicles lying beneath the smooth, glistening capsule are usually 10 to 12 mm in diameter.
   b. Polycystic ovary-derived granulosa cells are capable of the normal metabolism of androstenedione to estrogens.
   c. Polycystic ovary-derived granulosa cells have normal levels of the enzyme aromatase.
   d. Follicular fluid from polycystic ovaries have elevated levels of inhibin.

19–7. Which of the following statements is true regarding insulin resistance in PCOS?

   a. Patients with PCOS possess a specific post-receptor binding defect in insulin action.
   b. The normal insulin-induced tyrosine autophosphoryl relation is replaced by phosphoryl relation of serine.
   c. There is an impairment of insulin signal transduction.
   d. all of the above

19–8. Which of the following statements is NOT true regarding type A insulin-resistant patients?

   a. They are thin.
   b. Their disease manifests during the teenage years.
   c. Their disease entity may be either PCOS or hyperthecosis.
   d. They are more likely to manifest autoimmune disease than type B patients.

19–9. Which of the following statements is true regarding follicular fluid insulin levels?

   a. Insulin will not stimulate oocyte maturation in animal model systems.
   b. Insulin correlates with follicular progesterone and estradiol levels.
   c. Insulin correlates with follicular fluid androstenedione levels.
   d. Insulin has been identified in human follicular fluid, but it is unclear whether it is produced there or sequestered there.

19–10. Which of the following hormones is not elevated in PCOS?

   a. LH
   b. DHEAS
   c. ACTH
   d. androstenedione

19–11. Which of the following androgens is elevated in women with hyperprolactinemia?

   a. testosterone
   b. androstenedione
   c. DHEAS
   d. dihydrotestosterone (DHT)

19–12. Which of the following happens to the PCOS patient who reduces her body weight to less than 15 percent above ideal?

   a. There is a reduction in hyperinsulinemia.
   b. There is a reduction in insulin resistance.
   c. Gonadotropin and sex steroid secretion may be corrected.
   d. all of the above

19–13. The most common medication used in ovulation induction in the PCOS patient is

   a. bromocriptine
   b. dexamethasone
   c. clomiphene citrate
   d. human menopausal gonadotropin

19–14. Which of the following agents has been used to induce oocyte release?

   a. hCG 5000 units
   b. hCG 10,000 units
   c. 1 mg leuprolide acetate subcutaneously
   d. all of the above

19–15. Which of the following ovulation-induction protocols is most likely to yield monofollicular ovulation using purified FSH?

   a. a conventional high-dose fixed protocol
   b. a conventional increasing-dose protocol
   c. a decreasing-dose protocol
   d. a low, slow protocol

19–16. Which of the following statements is true regarding the ovarian wedge resection?

   a. It results in a high ovulation rate.
   b. It results in a pregnancy rate of approximately 68 percent.
   c. The effect diminishes after a year.
   d. all of the above

19–17. DHEAS is found to be elevated in PCOS patients what percentage of the time?

   a. 10 percent
   b. 20 percent
   c. 30 percent
   d. 50 percent

19–18. Hyperprolactinemia is said to be associated with PCOS what percentage of the time?

   a. 5 percent
   b. 10 percent
   c. 15 percent
   d. 20 percent

19–19. If sonography is used to diagnose PCOS, what percentage of women examined will have the disorder?

   a. 5 percent
   b. 10 percent
   c. 15 percent
   d. 22 percent

19–20. What is the prevalence of PCOS in women with ovulatory dysfunction?

   a. 50 percent
   b. 60 percent
   c. 70 percent
   d. 85 percent

19–21. Leptin is thought to alter hypothalamic GnRH secretion by acting through a release of

   a. thyrotropin-releasing hormone (TRH)
   b. neurotensin
   c. neuropeptide-Y
   d. serotonin

19–22. Which neurological disorder has been associated with PCOS?

   a. multiple sclerosis
   b. Niemann–Pick disease
   c. temporal lobe epilepsy
   d. Parkinson's disease

19–23. Which of the following conditions has been associated with ovarian hyperandrogenism?

   a. type A insulin resistance
   b. type B insulin resistance
   c. lipotropic diabetes
   d. all of the above

19–24. In anovulatory women with PCOS, high-density lipoprotein (HDL) does which of the following?

   a. decreases
   b. is unchanged
   c. increases
   d. the HDL/LDL (low-density lipoprotein) ratio is unchanged

19–25. Which of the following laboratory tests should be drawn when evaluating the patient with suspected PCOS?

   a. LH and FSH
   b. 17-OHP and DHEAS
   c. testosterone battery
   d. all of the above

19–26. Which of the following hormones is LEAST useful in evaluating the patient for PCOS?

   a. total testosterone
   b. free testosterone
   c. SHBG
   d. DHEAS

Chapter 20

HIRSUTISM AND VIRILISM

CASE REPORT

A 21-year-old nulliparous African-American woman with amenorrhea and severe virilization presented at Parkland Memorial Hospital. Postnatal and childhood growth and development were normal and there was no significant past history or family history. Growth spurt and pubertal development were normal; menarche occurred at age 13 and, thereafter, regular, cyclic, predictable menses occurred until age 19, at which time she experienced oligomenorrhea that lasted for 3 months followed by amenorrhea. She recounted the commencement of excess facial and body hair growth at age 17 that required daily shaving of beard and mustache 1 year later. Deepening of the voice, growth of the clitoris, increase in libido, and breast tissue loss were also present at that time.

She was 148 cm in height, weighed 47 kg, and exhibited a distinct male body habitus. Her blood pressure was 126/80 mm Hg, without postural changes. Facial and body hirsutism with temporal balding was evident (Fig 20–1A). Defeminization with loss of breast tissue and male muscular definition was present (Fig 20–1B). Her voice was moderately deep and husky; there was a male escutcheon; the clitoris was enlarged, 5 cm × 2 cm ×

1.5 cm (Fig 20–1C). The vagina was well rugated, pink, and moist. Cervical mucus was present. Neither adnexal nor abdominal masses were palpable, and the remainder of the physical examination was normal.

In a preliminary laboratory study, peripheral blood was collected and plasma was prepared and used to determine protein hormone, steroid, and electrolyte levels. By ultrasonography, there was an anteverted uterus (7 cm × 3.2 cm × 3 cm), right adnexa (3.2 cm × 2 cm × 3 cm), left adnexa (2 cm × 2 cm), and no abnormal masses. A tumor localized to the left adrenal gland was visualized by abdominal computerized axial tomography (CT) scan. The tumor was well circumscribed and without obvious invasion (Fig 20–2).

The results of a basal plasma hormone are presented in Table 20–1. Plasma levels of dehydroepiandrosterone (DHEA), dehydroepiandrosterone sulfate (DHEAS), androstenedione, 5-androstene-3β, 17β-diol, testosterone, and 5α-dihydrotestosterone were elevated 2- to 4-fold compared to normal women. The levels of the other hormones were not different from control women.

The patient underwent surgery with removal of a 90-g tan-white oval tumor (Fig 20–3). On histologic section, a well-circumscribed tumor compati-

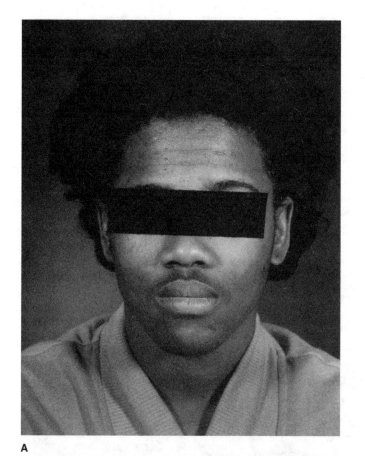

A

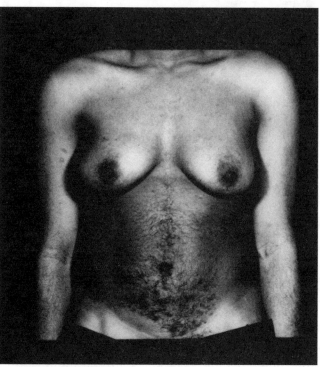

B

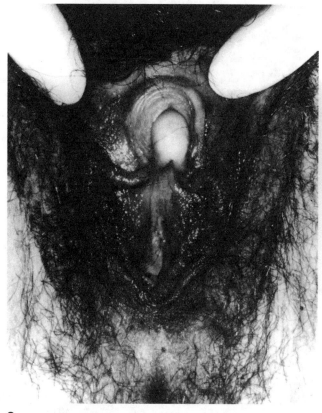

C

Figure 20–1. Clinical features of hirsutism and virilization in a woman with a virilizing adrenal adenoma. **A.** Photograph demonstrating facial hair and temporal balding. **B.** Photograph of the trunk and abdomen demonstrating muscle development and male escutcheon. **C.** Clitoromegaly. *(Courtesy of Dr. Karen D. Bradshaw, University of Texas Southwestern Medical Center at Dallas, Dallas, TX.) (From Carr BR. Disorders of the ovary and female reproductive tract. In: Wilson JD, Foster DW, eds. Williams Textbook of Endocrinology, 8th ed. Philadelphia, PA, W. B. Saunders, 1992: 733–798.*

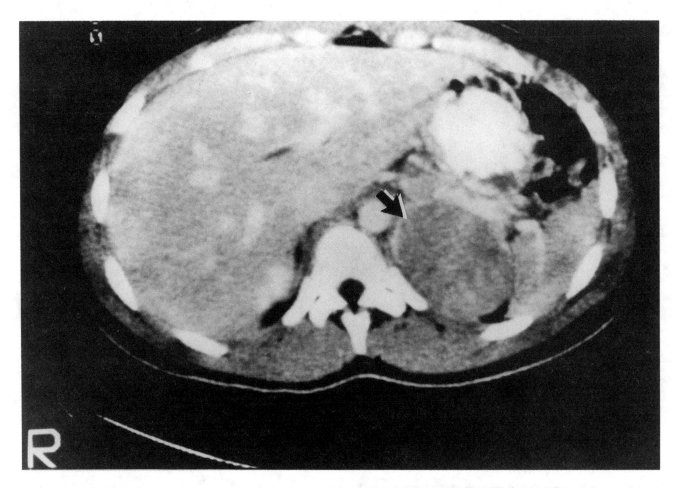

Figure 20–2. CT scan demonstrating an adrenal adenoma (arrow) of a woman with virilization (see Fig 20–1 for details). *(Courtesy of Dr. Karen D. Bradshaw, University of Texas Southwestern Medical Center at Dallas, Dallas, TX.) (From Carr BR. Disorders of the ovary and female reproductive tract. In: Wilson JD, Foster DW, eds.* Williams Textbook of Endocrinology, *8th ed. Philadelphia, PA, W. B. Saunders, 1992: 733–798.*

Table 20–1. Preoperative Plasma Hormone Levels in a Woman With a Virilizing Adenoma and in Normal Women

Hormone	Woman With Adrenal Adenoma	Normal Women
Follicle-stimulating hormone	4 IU/L	1.8–11.2 IU/L
Luteinizing hormone	11.6 IU/L	2–20 IU/L
Prolactin	7 µg/L	<20 µg/L
Dehydroepiandrosterone sulfate	36.9 µmol/L	2.2–9.2 µmol/L
Testosterone	2.8 nmol/L	0.03–1.9 nmol/L
Cortisol (pre-dexamethasone)	0.19 µmol/L	0.11–0.52 µmol/L
Cortisol (post-dexamethasone)	0.05 µmol/L	<0.14 µmol/L
17-Hydroxyprogesterone	7.9 nmol/L	1–13 nmol/L
Androstenedione	29.3 nmol/L	3–10.5 nmol/L
11-Desoxycortisol	3.5 nmol/L	<35 nmol/L
5α-Dihydrotestosterone	0.5 nmol/L	0.1–0.2 nmol/L
Dehydroepiandrosterone	19.1 nmol/L	4.8 nmol/L
5-Androstene-3β, 17β-diol	3.0 nmol/L	1.4 nmol/L

Reproduced, with permission, from Bradshaw KD, Milewich L, Mason JI, Parker CR Jr, MacDonald PC, Carr BR. Steroid secretory characteristics of a virilizing adenoma in a woman. *J Endocrinol.* 140:297, 1994.

ble with a histologic diagnosis of benign adrenal cortical adenoma was made.

Postoperatively, the plasma levels of DHEAS decreased to levels similar to those in normal women, whereas those of androstenedione, testosterone, 5α-dihydrotestosterone, DHEA, 5-androstene-3β, and 17β-estradiol (data not shown) decreased to levels even lower than those in normal women; cortisol levels, which were elevated on the day of surgery, were normal on the fourth and fifth days after surgery, but returned to levels found in normal women 14 days postoperatively. Approximately 6 weeks after extirpation of the tumor, the subject appeared to experience a slight reduction in the degree of hirsutism and male body contour, and menstruation occurred. Thirteen months after the removal of the tumor, this woman conceived and delivered a healthy female infant at term (by cesarean section). The subject was lost to follow-up 23 months after surgery.

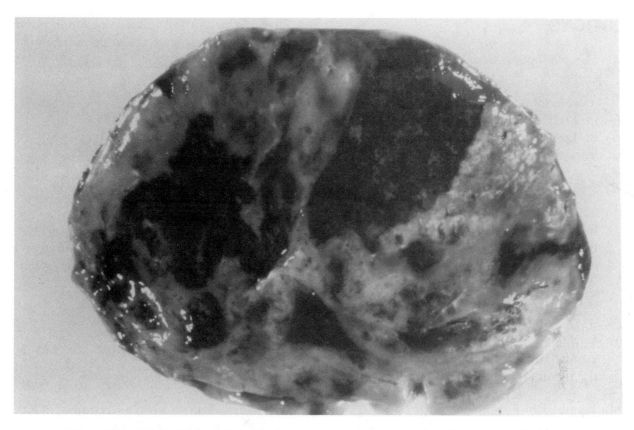

Figure 20–3. Gross tissue section of adrenal adenoma demonstrating significant hemorrhage. *(Courtesy of Dr. Karen D. Bradshaw, University of Texas Southwestern Medical Center at Dallas, Dallas, TX.)*

SUMMARY AND CONCLUSIONS

Benign adrenal adenomas are common in women and men. The incidence at autopsy studies is 2 percent (women) and 1 percent (men). Functioning adrenal adenomas that cause virilization in women without cortisol excess are extremely rare with less than 50 reported cases in the literature. The rapid onset of symptoms and signs of virilization suggested the presence of a tumor. Imaging studies including sonography, CT scans, or magnetic resonance imaging (MRI) are indicated to localize the tumor. The treatment is surgical, and rapid resolution of symptoms and virilization to varying degree as apparent in our subject is common.

BIBLIOGRAPHY

Bradshaw KD, Milewich L, Mason JI, Parker CR Jr, MacDonald PC, Carr BR. Steroid secretory characteristics of a virilizing adrenal adenoma in a woman. *J Endocrinol.* 140:297, 1994

Freeman DA. Steroid hormone-producing tumors in man. *Endocrine Rev.* 7:204, 1986

Gabrilove JL, Seaman AT, Sabet R, Mitty HA, Nicolis GL. Virilizing adrenal adenoma with studies of the steroid content of the adrenal venous effluent and a review of the literature. *Endocrine Rev.* 2:462, 1981

Munro-Neville A, O'Hare MJ. *The Human Adrenal Cortex—Pathology and Biology—An Integrated Approach.* New York, Springer-Verlag, 1982: 16–34

Russi S, Blumenthal HT, Gray SH. Small adenomas of the adrenal cortex in hypertension and diabetes. *Arch Int Med.* 76:284, 1945

CASE REPORT

QUESTIONS

20–1. Gonadotropin-releasing hormone (GnRH) analogs decrease the levels of

    a. cortisol
    b. DHEAS
    c. DHEA
    d. androstenedione

20–2. 3α-diol is a metabolite of

    a. testosterone
    b. 3α-hydroxysteroid dehydrogenase (HSD)
    c. 3β-HSD
    d. dihydrotestosterone

20–3. A normal level of testosterone in women is

    a. 0.5 ng/ml
    b. 5.0 ng/ml
    c. 50 ng/ml
    d. 500 ng/ml

20–4. Hypertrichosis is best defined as

    a. facial hair
    b. clitoromegaly
    c. generalized increase in body hair
    d. all of the above

20–5. Which of the following defines an abnormal clitoral index?

    a. >3.5 mm^2
    b. >35 mm^2
    c. >350 mm^2
    d. >500 mm^2

20–6. Which of the following medications is NOT associated with hirsutism?

    a. norethindrone
    b. levonorgestrel
    c. norgestimate
    d. danazol

20–7. Which of the following is associated with idiopathic hirsutism?

    a. normal menstrual cycles
    b. luteal-phase defects
    c. anovulation
    d. low estrogen levels

20–8. Which of the following ovarian tumors can secrete excessive androgen, leading to virilization?

    a. adrenal rest
    b. hilus cell
    c. Brenner tumor
    d. all of the above

20–9. Which of the following most likely supports the presence of an androgen-secreting tumor?

    a. DHEAS, 6 ng/ml
    b. testosterone, 1.6 ng/ml
    c. 17-hydroxyprogesterone (17-OHP), 100 pg/ml
    d. unilateral adnexal mass

20–10. A 24-year-old female develops increasing hirsutism, temporal balding, and deepening of the voice over a 3-year period. Which of the following is most likely?

    a. polycystic ovary syndrome (PCOS)
    b. adult-onset adrenal hyperplasia
    c. Sertoli–Leydig tumor
    d. all of the above

20–11. Adult-onset adrenal hyperplasia presents

    a. with a clinical presentation similar to PCOS
    b. in Ashkenazi Jews
    c. with elevated 17-OHP levels
    d. all of the above

20–12. Which of the following lowers serum androgen levels?

    a. 17α-estradiol
    b. ketoconazole
    c. desoxycorticosterone
    d. morphine

20–13. When finasteride is used as a treatment for hirsutism, which of the following describes its mechanisms or effects?

    a. inhibits 17α-hydroxylase
    b. inhibits 5α-reductase type I
    c. inhibits 5α-reductase type II
    d. lowers testosterone levels

20–14. Which of the following describes flutamide?

 a. nonsteroidal compound
 b. inhibits androgen action
 c. inhibits the androgen receptor
 d. all of the above

20–15. Which of the following is true for oral contraceptives in the treatment of hirsutism?

 a. lower DHEAS
 b. lower testosterone
 c. increase sex hormone-binding globulin (SHBG)
 d. all of the above

20–16. Adrenal virilizing adenomas are associated with

 a. increased cortisol levels
 b. familial history
 c. rapid progression of virilization
 d. postmenopausal women

20–17. Which of the following enzymes is present only in the adrenal?

 a. aromatase
 b. 17α-hydroxylase
 c. 11β-hydroxylase
 d. 3β-HSD

20–18. Which of the following defines virilization?

 a. excessive hair growth on hands
 b. excessive hair growth on legs
 c. increased muscle mass
 d. all of the above

20–19. Hyperthecosis includes which of the following?

 a. luteinized theca cells
 b. luteinizing hormone/follicle-stimulating hormone (LH/FSH) ratio >3:1
 c. responsive to clomiphene citrate (Clomid)
 d. all of the above

20–20. What percentage of estradiol is usually bound to SHBG?

 a. 10 percent
 b. 25 percent
 c. 35 percent
 d. 40 percent

20–21. The length of the anagen phase for scalp hair is

 a. 3 months
 b. 6 months
 c. 1 year
 d. 3 years

20–22. Which of the following factors causes hirsutism?

 a. danazol
 b. GnRH agonists
 c. desogestrel
 d. all of the above

20–23. Idiopathic hirsutism is associated with

 a. increased 3α-diol G
 b. positive family history
 c. increased 5α-reductase
 d. all of the above

20–24. PCOS is associated with all of the following EXCEPT

 a. LH/FSH ratio >2:1
 b. increased cortisol
 c. increased prolactin (PRL)
 d. decreased SHBG

20–25. Hilus cell tumors of the ovary are characterized by which of the following?

 a. usually detected by sonography
 b. secrete DHEAS
 c. secrete large amounts of testosterone
 d. comprise 30 percent of androgen-secreting tumors

20–26. Testosterone levels secreted by ovarian tumors are characterized by which of the following?

 a. levels usually >2 ng/ml
 b. suppressed by oral contraceptives
 c. suppressed by GnRH agonists
 d. all of the above

20–27. Spironolactone exhibits which of the following features?

 a. competitive inhibitor for androgen receptor
 b. inhibits 3β-HSD
 c. stimulates 17α-hydroxylase
 d. inhibits aromatase

21 ENDOCRINE ALTERATIONS IN FEMALE OBESITY

21–1. Body mass index is best defined as

a. height/weight
b. height/weight^2
c. weight/height
d. weight/height^2

21–2. Severe obesity is best defined as

a. >50 percent of ideal body weight
b. >100 percent of ideal body weight
c. >150 percent of ideal body weight
d. none of the above

21–3. Visceral fat is associated with

a. high apolipoprotein B (apo B) →↑LDL
b. large low-density lipoprotein (LDL) particle size
c. small high-density lipoprotein (HDL) particle size
d. all of the above

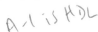

21–4. The metabolic clearance of which of the following hormones is NOT increased in obese women?

a. dehydroepiandrosterone (DHEA)
b. testosterone
c. dihydrotestosterone
d. 3α-androstenedione

21–5. What percentage of circulating androstenedione is converted to estrone?

a. 0
b. 5 percent
c. 10.5 percent
d. 15 percent

21–6. Metformin exhibits which of the following in polycystic ovary syndrome (PCOS)?

a. results in ovulatory rates of 30 to 50 percent
b. increases insulin levels
c. inhibits follicle-stimulating hormone (FSH) levels
d. inhibits luteinizing hormone (LH) levels

21–7. In obese postmenopausal women, which of the following is correct?

a. increased sex hormone-binding globulin (SHBG)
b. decreased free estradiol (E_2) levels
c. low estrone levels
d. none of the above

21–8. In obese women, estrone is metabolized to a greater degree to

a. estriol
b. catechol estrogen
c. estradiol
d. none of the above

21–9. The increase in production rate of estrogen in obese women occurs primarily by conversion of

a. testosterone
b. androstenedione
c. DHEA
d. all of the above

21–10. SHBG levels are increased by

    a. androgen
    b. cortisol
    c. estrogen
    d. progesterone

21–11. After the menopause, women deposit fat in which primary region?

    a. gluteal
    b. abdominal
    c. visceral
    d. all of the above

21–12. Growth hormone (GH) in obese women is associated with

    a. increased secretion
    b. increased clearance
    c. increased levels in the blood
    d. all of the above

21–13. Leptin is characterized by which of the following?

    a. It is a hormone.
    b. It is secreted by adipocytes.
    c. It promotes satiety.
    d. all of the above

21–14. Which of the following is true for obese premenopausal women in regard to gonadotropins compared to results in normal-weight women?

    a. LH basal levels are increased.
    b. FSH levels are similar.
    c. LH pulsatility is increased.
    d. all of the above

21–15. Obesity in women is associated with all of the following EXCEPT

    a. delayed menarche
    b. increased risk of anovulation
    c. increased risk of menorrhagia
    d. low levels of GH

21–16. Which of the following is true in obese eumenorrheic women compared to normal-weight eumenorrheic women?

    a. higher metabolic clearance rate (MCR) for androstenedione
    b. higher production rate (PR) for DHEA
    c. no difference in integrated plasma concentration of androstenedione
    d. all of the above

21–17. Which of the following is true regarding obese women compared to normal-weight women?

    a. Obese women have higher prolactin.
    b. Obese women have an increased rate of conversion of androstenedione to estrone.
    c. Obese women have a decreased rate of conversion of androstenedione to testosterone.
    d. all of the above

21–18. Which of the following is NOT true regarding obesity?

    a. Obese prepubertal girls have delayed menarche.
    b. Obese girls have accelerated linear growth.
    c. Obese women have higher insulin levels.
    d. Obese women have higher insulin-like growth factor I (IGF-I) levels.

21–19. All of the following are risk factors for endometrial carcinoma EXCEPT

    a. age at first pregnancy
    b. obesity (total body weight)
    c. anovulatory cycles
    d. insulin-resistant diabetes

21–20. Breast cancer is associated with increased fat in which of the following areas?

    a. proximal
    b. central
    c. distal
    d. all of the above

21–21. GH has been shown to exhibit which of the following effects on ovarian function?

    a. increased estrogen, increased progesterone
    b. increased estrogen, lower progesterone
    c. lower estrogen, increased progesterone
    d. lower estrogen, lower progesterone

21–22. Which of the following is NOT true regarding SHBG and obesity?

    a. decreased levels in obese women
    b. high-fat diet increases SHBG
    c. weight loss increases SHBG
    d. decreased levels in insulin-resistant diabetes

21–23. SHBG is

    a. β-globulin
    b. α-globulin
    c. Δ-globulin
    d. none of the above

21–24. Which of the following is a catechol estrogen?

    a. estradiol glucuronide
    b. estriol

    c. 2-hydroxyesterone
    d. estrone

21–25. Which of the following serves as the major substrate for estrone production formed outside the ovary?

    a. 17β-estradiol
    b. testosterone
    c. androsterone
    d. androstenedione

21–26. What percentage of E_2 is converted to estrone (E_1) in premenopausal women?

    a. 0.15 percent
    b. 1.5 percent
    c. 15 percent
    d. none of the above

21–27. Peripheral aromatization of androgens is positively associated with all of the following EXCEPT

    a. increasing body weight
    b. growth hormone level
    c. increasing age
    d. number of fat cells

22

Chapter 22

BREAST DISEASE

CASE REPORT

The patient is a 44-year-old white female who was first seen at age 35 in 1988 for the treatment of endometriosis diagnosed by laparoscopy in 1976. She had 4 months of increasing dysmenorrhea and pain with bowel movements and urination. Sonar and computed tomography (CT) scan showed a right adnexal mass of 4.5 cm. She underwent operative laparoscopy with resection of bilateral endometriomas and lysis of adhesions.

The patient was diagnosed in July 1988 with a left breast mass. This was subsequently evaluated at University Medical Center, and she underwent a left modified radical mastectomy and biopsy of the right breast. The tumor type was an interductal papillary carcinoma, the nodes were negative, and the tumor was positive for both estrogen and progesterone receptors. She was followed conservatively from the point of view of her endometriosis; however, in September 1991, she was found to have a 4-cm right ovarian cyst (Table 22–1). In October 1991, the cystic structure was found to be 2.2 × 5.5 × 6.5 cm. She also had a smaller cystic structure (1.7 × 2.2 × 1.1 cm) on the left ovary. Follow-up scan one month later confirmed the presence of the masses.

She underwent an operative laparoscopy in November 1991, with the finding of a large right endometrioma, a small left endometrioma, adhesions involving the left fallopian tube, and endometriosis implants on the bladder and uterosacral ligament, with a revised American Fertility Society (AFS) classification score of 26. These lesions were all treated at that juncture with operative laparoscopy.

Subsequently, the patient was begun on tamoxifen therapy at 10 mg b.i.d. as part of an oncology research protocol. In January 1993, she was found to have a metastasis with an ill-defined 5-mm lesion of the right lung. In February 1993, the patient complained of the development of lower abdominal pain during the last few cycles, particularly on the left side. Examination showed no ovarian enlargement. Two months later the patient developed a spontaneous right-sided pneumothorax; following her recovery in August 1993, a CT scan of the chest showed a stable right upper lobe nodule in the face of the tamoxifen therapy. Baseline sonar scan at that time showed a 0.9-cm trilaminar endometrium and normal right and left ovaries.

Unfortunately, in January 1994, the patient presented with left-sided pain. Sonar scan showed a 3.5 cm clear cyst with free fluid. The endometrium

Table 22–1. Flow Diagram of Treatment and Symptoms of Patient With Breast Cancer

Date	Symptoms	Medications	Sonar
1/93	Asymptomatic	Tamoxifen begun	
2/93	Left lower quadrant pain		Sonar negative
8/93	Asymptomatic		Normal ovaries; 0.9-cm endometrium
1/94	Left lower quadrant pain		3.5-cm left cystic ovary, free fluid; 1.0-cm endometrium with bleeding
6/94	Pain, bleeding	Lupron, 3.75 mg	Endometrium increased to 1.4 cm; 3.75-cm left cyst
7/94	Asymptomatic	Lupron, 3.75 mg × 2 months	0.8-cm endometrium; left ovary 1.7 × 2.2 × 1.2 cm; right ovary 3.3 × 2.3 × 2.3 cm
8/94	Asymptomatic		0.6-cm endometrium; right ovary 2.8 × 2.1 × 1.7 cm; left ovary 2.2 × 3.0 × 2.4 cm

97

was 1 cm, and she had persisted in having irregular bleeding. Follow-up evaluation in June 1994 showed a 1.4-cm endometrium with a residual ovarian cyst. Leuprolide acetate (Lupron), 3.75 mg, was administered at this juncture. A repeat scan done in July 1994 showed a 0.8-cm endometrium with normal-sized ovaries—1.7 × 2.2 × 1.2 cm on the left, and 3.3 × 2.3 × 2.3 cm on the right. In view of her history of stage III endometriosis, it was elected to continue co-therapy with Lupron for 2 further months. A scan done in August 1994 showed a 0.6-cm endometrium with ovaries measuring 2.8 × 2.1 × 1.7 cm on the right and 2.2 × 3.0 × 2.4 cm on the left. The patient was continued on her tamoxifen therapy throughout the Lupron suppression, which controlled both her pain and irregular bleeding.

SUMMARY AND CONCLUSIONS

Tamoxifen, when first introduced into the market, was widely used for the adjunctive treatment of breast cancer in postmenopausal patients. Today, premenopausal patients are being treated with tamoxifen with the same enthusiasm. Unfortunately, the gynecologic consequences of this form of therapy went unnoted until it was discovered that a few patients rapidly developed well-differentiated endometrial cancers in association with this treatment. This should in fact come as no surprise, as tamoxifen is quite similar to drugs such as clomiphene citrate. These agents act as both estrogen agonists and antagonists; that is, they antagonize the biological effect of 17β-estradiol, yet have endogenous estrogen activities of their own. All patients that we have seen managed with tamoxifen therapy who are premenopausal have developed thickened endometria, bleeding, pain, and large ovarian cysts. We have treated each of these problems with the co-administration of Depo-Lupron, 3.75 mg, and in all cases the ovarian cysts have resolved and endometrium returned to less than 1 cm in thickness within 1 to 2 months of therapy. This form of suppressive therapy can be used without disrupting tamoxifen administration.

BIBLIOGRAPHY

Dupont WD. Evidence of efficacy of mammographic screening for women in their forties. *Cancer.* 74:1204, 1994

Futreal PA, Liu Q, Shattuck-Eldens D, et al. BRAC1 mutations in primary breast and ovarian carcinomas. *Science.* 266:120, 1994

Molitch M, Elton R, Blackwell RE, et al, and the Bromocriptine Study Group. Bromocriptine as primary therapy for prolactin secreting macroadenomas: results of a prospective, multicenter study. *J Clin Endocrinol Metab.* 60(4):698, 1985

Wooster R, Neuhausen SL, Mangion J, et al. Localization of a breast cancer gene. BRAC2 to chromosome 13q12–13. *Science.* 265:2088, 1994

Zhang S, Folsom AR, Sellers TA, et al. Better breast cancer survival for postmenopausal women who are less overweight and eat less fat. *Cancer.* 76:275, 1995

QUESTIONS

22–1. Which of the following is true regarding nipple inversion?

    a. It is an uncommon condition that is not rectified by cosmetic surgery.

    b. Nipple inversion does not resolve during pregnancy.

    c. Cosmetic repair of nipple inversion may produce difficulty with breast feeding.

    d. Bilateral nipple inversion is not a sign of malignancy.

22–2. Breast hypertrophy may be associated with

    a. chest wall and shoulder pain

    b. image distortion

    c. intense sexual pressure

    d. all of the above

22–3. Which of the following breast infections is associated with a greenish discharge?

    a. *Staphylococcus*

    b. *Pseudomonas*

    c. *Streptococcus*

    d. *Escherichia coli*

22–4. Which of the following is NOT true regarding galactoceles?

    a. They occur secondary to mechanical duct obstruction.

    b. Pressure can often result in emptying of the lesion.

    c. Galactoceles can calcify.

    d. Fluid drawn from a galactocele tends to be green to yellow-green and usually contains bacteria.

22–5. Which of the following does NOT describe mammary dysplasia?

   a. It could be bilateral or unilateral.
   b. It is frequently seen in the lower inner quadrant.
   c. The disorder exacerbates during menstruation.
   d. It usually resolves after menopause.

22–6. The interductal papilloma is a benign lesion of the lactiferous duct wall that usually occurs below the areola what percentage of the time?

   a. 10 percent
   b. 75 percent
   c. 25 percent
   d. 50 percent

22–7. Which of the following is NOT true with regard to fibroadenomas?

   a. The lesions are multiple 20 percent of the time.
   b. The lesions may be painful and hormonally responsive.
   c. The lesions occur more commonly in whites than blacks.
   d. These lesions are not associated with an increased risk of carcinoma.

22–8. Which of the following best describes the screening mammography?

   a. Baseline examination should be obtained by 40 years of age.
   b. In the face of a positive family history, examination should be performed yearly.
   c. Mammograms should be performed yearly in women 50 years of age and older.
   d. all of the above

22–9. Which of the following is true regarding carcinoma of the breast?

   a. The stage or presentation is not related to income.
   b. There is no relationship between ethnicity and the incidence of lower-stage disease.

   c. There is no regional variation in terms of early-stage disease presentation.
   d. There is marked regional variation in the use of partial mastectomy.

22–10. Which of the following are risk factors for breast cancer?

   a. positive family history
   b. failure to give birth before age 35
   c. smoking, high-fat diet, and alcohol intake
   d. all of the above

22–11. Which of the following is true with regard to tamoxifen?

   a. It is an estrogen antagonist.
   b. It is effective in postmenopausal women with positive nodes who are receptor negative.
   c. It results in endometrial hypoplasia.
   d. Adenocarcinomas of the uterus have not been detected with the use of this drug.

22–12. Women who consume more than three alcoholic drinks a day have what percentage increase in the risk of breast cancer?

   a. 10 percent
   b. 20 percent
   c. 30 percent
   d. 40 percent

22–13. Which of the following best describes the genetics of breast cancer?

   a. There appears to be a two- to threefold increased incidence in women who have a female relative with the disease.
   b. If a patient's mother is affected, there is a 2.3 percent increased relative risk of developing breast cancer.
   c. Hereditary forms of breast cancer make up 8 percent of the disease.
   d. all of the above

22–14. Which of the following genes is associated with both an increased incidence of breast cancer and ovarian cancer?

    a. BRAC2
    b. BRAC1
    c. RAS
    d. BAM

22–15. Which of the following breast lesions is premalignant?

    a. interductal papilloma
    b. fibroadenoma
    c. adenosis
    d. florid sclerosing adenosis

22–16. Which of the following agents has been used to treat mastodynia?

    a. cyclic analgesics or nonsteroidal anti-inflammatory drugs (NSAIDs)
    b. monophasic oral contraceptive agents
    c. low-dose danazol
    d. all of the above

22–17. Polythelia occurs in what percentage of the population?

    a. 1 to 2 percent
    b. 3 to 5 percent
    c. 7 percent
    d. 9 percent

22–18. Which of the following denotes multiple nipples?

    a. athelia
    b. polymastia
    c. amastia
    d. polyathelia

22–19. In the condition premature thelarche, serum gonadotropin levels show which of the following patterns?

    a. hypogonadotropic
    b. prepubertal
    c. adult cycling
    d. elevated levels

22–20. Which of the following is associated with breast hypoplasia?

    a. hypothalamic amenorrhea as associated with eating disorders
    b. patients with selective gonadotropin deficiencies
    c. women taking gonadotropin-releasing hormone (GnRH) analogs
    d. all of the above

22–21. Which of the following is the most serious consequence of breast augmentation procedures?

    a. complicates self-examination process
    b. increases difficulty of the radiographic surveillance for malignancies
    c. interferes with breast feeding
    d. implants may become dislocated or leak

22–22. Which of the following will be found on microscopic examination of breast discharge from a woman with simple galactorrhea?

    a. acellular green/gray fluid
    b. squamous cells
    c. fat globules
    d. rod-like bacteria

22–23. Which of the following amino acids has NOT been shown to release prolactin (PRL) under special circumstances?

    a. tyrosine
    b. tryptophan
    c. arginine
    d. glycine

22–24. Which of the following best describes the kinetics of vaginal PRL metabolism?

    a. Serum levels rise slower than with oral administration but remain elevated longer.
    b. Serum levels rise more rapidly than with oral administration and remain elevated longer.

c. Serum levels rise at the same rate as oral administration yet remain elevated longer.

d. Serum levels rise slower than with oral administration yet decrease more rapidly.

22–25. Which of the following antihyperprolactinemic drugs available in Europe has just been introduced into the U.S. market?

a. Norprolac
b. Parlodel SRO
c. Parlodel LAR
d. Dostinex (cabergoline)

22–26. Which of the following agents has been used to treat mastodynia?

a. Danocrine (danazol)
b. GnRH analogs
c. Aygestin (norethindrone acetate)
d. all of the above

Chapter 23

PSYCHOLOGICAL ASPECTS OF MENSTRUATION: PREMENSTRUAL SYNDROME

23–1. The term used to describe late luteal symptoms of mild severity that are experienced by most women is

    a. premenstrual tension
    b. premenstrual syndrome (PMS)
    c. premenstrual molimina
    d. all of the above

23–2. To differentiate PMS from other mood disorders, which of the following is required?

    a. There is at least 1 week during the follicular phase in which the patient is asymptomatic.
    b. The patient is usually asymptomatic during the menses.
    c. The patient may develop symptoms at midcycle (day of ovulation).
    d. all of the above

23–3. Which of the following is a useful symptom record for rapid visual confirmation of PMS?

    a. PMDD
    b. PRISM
    c. MPSD
    d. none of the above

23–4. What percentage of reproductive women with premenstrual symptoms are categorized as severe and temporarily disabling?

    a. 80 percent
    b. 60 percent
    c. 10 percent
    d. 5 percent

23–5. Which of the following is true regarding PMS?

    a. Severe, disabling PMS occurs in 10 percent of women.
    b. Symptoms are improved with phasic oral contraceptives.
    c. It is rare in breast-feeding women.
    d. none of the above

23–6. Which of the following is NOT true regarding PMS?

    a. It does not worsen after pregnancy.
    b. It increases after tubal ligation.
    c. Genetic factors are not involved in the etiology.
    d. It is commonly associated with dysmenorrhea.

23–7. Which of the following confirms the association of bloating or swelling in women experiencing PMS?

    a. documented weight gain of 3 to 5 lb
    b. increase in total body water
    c. associated with local fluid shifts
    d. all of the above

23–8. Which of the following medical conditions worsens during the late luteal or menstrual phase of the cycle?

   a. asthma
   b. epilepsy
   c. arthritis
   d. all of the above

23–9. Which of the following is true regarding the association of PMS and vitamin deficiency or treatment?

   a. Vitamin B_6 deficiency causes PMS.
   b. Vitamin B_6 therapy may cause neuropathy.
   c. Vitamin A improves PMS.
   d. Vitamin E may improve PMS.

23–10. Which of the following hormone changes may be associated with PMS?

   a. progesterone deficiency
   b. estrogen excess
   c. serotonin deficiency
   d. norepinephrine deficiency

23–11. Which of the following is true regarding PMS?

   a. rare before menarche
   b. rare after menopause
   c. persists following total abdominal hysterectomy
   d. all of the above

23–12. Which of the following life-style modifications does NOT benefit PMS?

   a. diets
   b. exercising
   c. decreased caffeine intake
   d. none of the above

23–13. Premenstrual mastalgia responds to all of the following EXCEPT

   a. pyridoxine
   b. tamoxifen
   c. bromocriptine
   d. danazol

23–14. Which of the following treatments of PMS yields the best results?

   a. oral contraceptives
   b. progesterone suppositories
   c. danazol
   d. micronized progesterone

23–15. Which of the following therapies may offer excellent results for depression associated with PMS?

   a. fluoxetine
   b. reserpine
   c. serotonin
   d. micronized progesterone

23–16. Which of the following biochemical tests is diagnostic of PMS?

   a. progesterone
   b. estrogen
   c. β-endorphin
   d. none of the above

23–17. All of the following parameters must be evaluated in establishing the diagnosis of PMS EXCEPT

   a. nature of symptoms
   b. severity of symptoms
   c. frequency of symptoms during menstruation
   d. timing of symptoms in relation to menstruation

23–18. Which of the following does NOT describe the four temporal patterns of symptoms of PMS?

   a. increases last half of cycle
   b. decreases on day 10 of cycle
   c. decreases on last day of menses
   d. peak seen at midcycle (ovulation)

23–19. Which of the following terms is utilized by the American Psychiatric Association to describe PMS?

   a. PMDD
   b. PRISM
   c. MPSD
   d. none of the above

23–20. What percentage of women of reproductive age experience some temporary distress each month related to premenstrual symptomatology?

    a. 95 percent
    b. 75 percent
    c. 30 percent
    d. 10 percent

23–21. Which of the following is true regarding PMS?

    a. occurs only in Western cultures
    b. absent in Japanese women
    c. absent in subhuman primates
    d. none of the above

23–22. Which of the following is true regarding PMS?

    a. onset usually occurs at menarche
    b. usually appears suddenly and without warning
    c. can disappear suddenly without treatment or intervention
    d. none of the above

23–23. Which of the following is true regarding PMS and legal issues in the United States?

    a. Cases of child abuse are often excused in PMS mothers.
    b. Murder of spouse may be excused in women with PMS.
    c. Legal experts rarely introduce PMS into courts.
    d. PMS has no legal basis.

23–24. Which of the following is true regarding PMS and thyroid function?

    a. thyroid-stimulating hormone (TSH) increases
    b. thyroxine-binding globulin (TBG) decreases
    c. free triiodothyronine (T_3) decreases
    d. none of the above

23–25. Which of the following are plausible cases of PMS?

    a. bacterial
    b. candidal
    c. serotonin deficiency
    d. none of the above

23–26. PMS improves with which of the following treatments in double-blind, controlled studies?

    a. evening primrose oil (EPO)
    b. vitamin B_{12}
    c. mifepristone (RU 486)
    d. doxycycline

23–27. Which of the following is considered a "second"-level intervention?

    a. pyridoxine
    b. bromocriptine
    c. gonadotropin-releasing hormone (GnRH) agonists
    d. mefenamic acid

Chapter 24

CHRONIC PELVIC PAIN: ORIGIN, PHYSIOLOGY, EVALUATION, AND TREATMENT

CASE REPORT

The patient is an 18-year-old white female, para 0-0-0-0, with a history positive for both endometriosis and chronic pelvic pain (Fig 24–1). Menarche occurred at age 14, and she began to have progressive dysmenorrhea that was incapacitating. The pelvic pain became so severe that she was unable to work. Her episodes of dysmenorrhea were associated with protracted nausea, vomiting, and diarrhea; she has had multiple admissions for rehydration and has been evaluated by the university gastroenterology service. At the time of her first office visit she was being managed by her family physician, using a home health service with intravenous (IV) fluid therapy, as well as meperidine (Demerol) and promethazine (Phenergan). She also used Tylox, Toradol, and Anaprox, each of which gave some pain relief but exacerbated the problem of recurrent vomiting. She had become quite thin, losing approximately 10 lb over the last year. Her gastroenterology workup had included a colonoscopy, abdominal CT scan, and abdominal ultrasound, all which were negative. She had undergone a laparoscopy with presacral neurectomy, which resulted in no relief of her symptoms. She claimed not to be sexually active but had been treated with contraceptive agents as well as Depo-Provera in the past without relief.

Her past medical history was significant in that she had undergone a cholecystectomy, yet the tissue specimen was negative for disease at the time of evaluation. The patient is single, lives with her mother and father, is a high school graduate, and is currently unemployed secondary to the severe pain. She denies smoking or using alcohol or recreational drugs.

Physical examination showed the following: height, 5'8"; weight, 92 lb; blood pressure, 110/66; pulse, 70; skin, no abnormalities; HEENT, benign; neck, no thyromegaly; chest, clear; heart, regular sinus rhythm without murmurs; breasts, Tanner stage V, no discharge or mass present; and pelvic, negative. Her admitting diagnosis was severe endometriosis, chronic pelvic pain syndrome, and probable addiction to narcotics.

She was initially treated with Depo-Lupron, 3.75 mg, and a limited supply of hydrocodone suppositories and Phenergan suppositories. Hydrocodone was chosen secondary to intractable nausea and vomiting and the wish to avoid IV therapy if necessary. Discussion was carried out with the patient and her mother about the possible need for addiction treatment as well as psychological counseling. Further consultation was obtained from the gastroenterology service and bariatrics group as well as the drug addiction service and adolescent psychiatry. The idea of self-induced vomiting was entertained, and it was felt that with her current

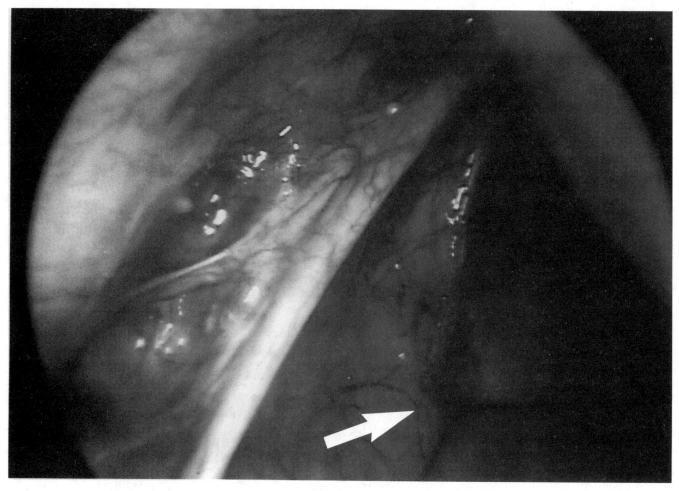

Figure 24–1. Laparoscopic image of left uterosacral ligament and pelvic floor with typical and atypical endometriosis involving the peritoneum in a patient with chronic pelvic pain.

weight of 92 lb and height of 5'8", she was functioning as an individual who really had an eating disorder and would probably develop a state of secondary amenorrhea that would biologically control active endometriosis and eliminate menses and dysmenorrhea. Unfortunately, depression was thought to be part of her problem, which would be aggravated in this anorectic, bulimic-type cycle.

The patient was seen in follow-up approximately 3 weeks after her initial consultation. Her weight had remained stable, she was able to eat some food without vomiting, and she was begun on a program to wean her from narcotics. Her pain medication was reduced to Darvocet-M 100; however, before leaving the office, the patient's mother indicated that she felt her daughter needed to be continued on narcotics as she was sure she would become nauseated on the way home. One week

later the patient's primary doctor called, saying that she was having nausea and vomiting and that she was being placed on IV home therapy again with Phenergan and narcotics. At this juncture, the patient was admitted to the university hospital gynecological service, and consultation was obtained with the drug addiction service. She was begun on a detoxification program, which met with considerable resistance. She was placed on a low-dose Demerol PCA (patient-controlled analgesia) pump in an ever-progressing tapering dose over a week, and was treated with intravenous gramisetron (Kytril) to control her nausea.

Subsequently, a series of consultations was undertaken with her mother, which revealed a pertinent social history. Immediately prior to the onset of the patient's original abdominal pain some 2 years before, her parents learned that she was sexually active, and the relationship with her boyfriend was terminated by the family. She had experienced the death of several family members who were close to her, and her brother remarried and he and his wife had a child. The mother states that they were afraid to leave the daughter with the child for fear she would harm it. The first episode of vomiting, which ultimately resulted in her cholecystectomy, occurred several days before she was due to enter college. Her mother further stated that the daughter appeared to be able to control the vomiting—when entering a vomiting episode, if she became angry, she would actually voluntarily stop and leave the house.

From this additional history it became apparent that we were dealing with a dysfunctional family relationship. It should be noted that, despite the hospitalization, the father never accompanied the mother or daughter to the office for consultation and was never seen in the hospital. Subsequently, despite considerable protest from the daughter, she was admitted to the adolescent psychiatry unit, was isolated from the family for several weeks, and finally withdrawn from all IV therapy. The mother and father agreed to enter into a family counseling arrangement, and the patient was discharged from the hospital approximately 3 weeks after her original admission to the reproductive endocrine service.

SUMMARY AND CONCLUSIONS

This case represents many important issues with regard to chronic pelvic pain. First of all, in terms of pathophysiologic factors, this patient's condition was poorly defined in terms of peripheral nociceptive mechanisms. While in fact having stage I endometriosis, this patient underwent a cholecystectomy, laparoscopy, and presacral neurectomy as a result of the symptom complex. Many psychological factors were obviously at play. She assumed the sick role, had a very aberrant behavior regarding her illness, achieved secondary gain by manipulating her family and health care providers, and had a significant depressive component to her problem as well as some element of antisocial personality. The therapeutic implications of this case show that anti-inflammatory agents are very unlikely to be effective. Narcotics as well as sedative hypnotics are contraindicated, yet this patient developed a drug addiction problem. Antidepressants would have been useful and were finally employed following admission to the adolescent psychiatry service, improving her coping strategies. Had neural blockade been attempted to relieve her pain, the response would have been unpredictable and would usually have been ineffective.

BIBLIOGRAPHY

Bonica JJ. General considerations of chronic pain. In: Bonica JJ (ed). *The Management of Pain.* Philadelphia, PA, Lea & Febiger, 1990: 180

Donnez J, Nisolle M, Somes P, Gillett N, et al. Peritoneal endometriosis and "endometriotic" nodules of the rectovaginal septum are two different entities. *Fertil Steril.* 66:361, 1996

Katon W, Lin E, Von Korff M, et al. Somatization: a spectrum of severity. *Am J Psychiatry.* 148:34, 1991

Koziol JA, Clark DC, Gittes RF, et al. The natural history of interstitial cystitis: a survey of 374 patients. *J Urol.* 149:465, 1993

Melzack R, Wall PD. Pain mechanisms: a new theory. *Science.* 150:971, 1978

Rapkin AJ, Mayer EA. Gastroenterologic causes of chronic pelvic pain. *Obstet Gynecol Clin North Am.* 20:663, 1993

QUESTIONS

24–1. The hallmark of chronic pelvic pain syndrome is best described by which of the following statements?

   a. The symptoms are always restricted to the pelvis.

   b. Social factors play a minor part in the syndrome.

   c. Polydrug abuse is rarely found in these patients.

   d. The patient's condition is poorly defined in terms of peripheral nociceptive mechanisms.

24–2. Which of the following is a psychological factor associated with chronic pain syndrome?

   a. depression

   b. sick role

   c. drug dependence

   d. all of the above

24–3. Which of the following social factors is associated with chronic pain syndrome?

    a. history of sexual abuse
    b. secondary gain
    c. family dysfunction
    d. all of the above

24–4. Patients with chronic pelvic pain syndrome frequently demonstrate all of the following EXCEPT

    a. polydrug dependence
    b. depression
    c. normal affect
    d. family dysfunction

24–5. Which of the following best defines pain?

    a. It may be point specific or very diffuse.
    b. It may be intermittent or continuous.
    c. It may be related to activity or exercise.
    d. all of the above

24–6. Which of the following neurochemicals is NOT a mediator of pain?

    a. substance P
    b. serotonin
    c. thyrotropin-releasing hormone (TRH)
    d. bradykinin

24–7. Which of the following statements is NOT true regarding nociceptors?

    a. They function in a proportional manner.
    b. Once a receptor is activated, a state of hyperalgesia is achieved.
    c. Nociceptors have been identified in all visceral tissue.
    d. There are more nociceptors in the viscera than in the skin.

24–8. Which of the following stimuli is more likely to produce pain?

    a. cutting a mesentery
    b. burning a mesentery
    c. touching a mesentery
    d. placing traction on a mesentery

24–9. Which of the following is NOT true regarding nociceptors?

    a. They are free nerve endings that respond to noxious stimuli.
    b. The receptors may be of high-intensity, thermal, chemical, or mechanical types
    c. The signaling is mediated by A-Δ and C-afferent fibers.
    d. Receptors are modality nonspecific.

24–10. Which of the following neurochemicals is thought to inhibit primary afferent transmission?

    a. vasoactive intestinal peptide (VIP)
    b. somatostatin
    c. enkephalins
    d. glycine

24–11. In the classic gate theory proposed by Melzac and Wall, which of the following neurotransmitters is the principal mediator of the process?

    a. gamma-aminobutyric acid (GABA)
    b. neurotensin
    c. somatostatin
    d. VIP

24–12. Which of the following chemical compounds does NOT cause constipation?

    a. opiates
    b. calcium channel blockers
    c. theophylline
    d. barium sulfate

24–13. Which of the following medical conditions is associated with chronic constipation?

    a. hypothyroidism
    b. Parkinson's disease
    c. multiple sclerosis
    d. all of the above

24–14. Which of the following is thought to be associated with interstitial cystitis?

    a. autoimmune reactions
    b. mast cell infiltrates
    c. urinary toxins
    d. all of the above

24–15. Which of the following is a symptom of endometriosis?

 a. medial thigh pain
 b. cyclic dyschezia
 c. cyclic dysuria
 d. all of the above

24–16. Which of the following drugs can induce diarrhea?

 a. alcohol
 b. nonsteroidal anti-inflammatory drugs (NSAIDs)
 c. theophylline
 d. all of the above

24–17. Malabsorption is associated with

 a. hyperthyroidism
 b. diabetes
 c. Zollinger–Ellison syndrome
 d. all of the above

24–18. Which condition is found 50 percent of the time in individuals over age 65 with pain and constipation?

 a. diverticular disease
 b. multiple sclerosis
 c. Parkinson's disease
 d. hypothyroidism

24–19. Vague abdominal pain, bloating, and bowel dysfunction are characteristic of

 a. irritable bowel syndrome
 b. diabetes
 c. Crohn's disease
 d. short bowel syndrome

24–20. Conditions that mimic interstitial cystitis include

 a. urethral syndrome
 b. irritable bladder syndrome
 c. sensory neuropathic urgency
 d. all of the above

24–21. Which of the following is a symptom of interstitial cystitis?

 a. urinary frequency
 b. urgency
 c. urethral and bladder pain
 d. all of the above

24–22. The incidence of interstitial cystitis is what percentage per 100,000 women?

 a. 1.2 percent
 b. 2.5 percent
 c. 4 percent
 d. 7 percent

24–23. Which of the following medications has been used to treat interstitial cystitis by bladder installation?

 a. dimethyl sulfoxide (DMSO)
 b. heparin
 c. silver nitrate
 d. all of the above

24–24. Which of the following drugs with its anticholinergic, antihistaminic, analgesic, and antidepressive effects has proven useful in treating interstitial cystitis?

 a. nifedipine
 b. glucocorticoids
 c. local anesthetics
 d. amitriptyline

24–25. Which of the following has been shown to be useful in the treatment of irritable bowel syndrome?

 a. bran and other bulk agents
 b. antispasmodics
 c. tranquilizers
 d. all of the above

24–26. Which of the following agents has been used to treat Crohn's disease?

 a. azathioprine
 b. methotrexate
 c. cyclosporine
 d. all of the above

V

INFERTILITY

25 CLINICAL TRIALS FOR THE REPRODUCTIVE ENDOCRINOLOGIST: DESIGN, POWER ANALYSIS, AND BIOSTATISTICS

25–1. Which of the following trials would be best to evaluate the efficacy of a new contraceptive agent?

   a. retrospective trial
   b. prospective, randomized clinical trial
   c. cohort study
   d. none of the above

25–2. The basic components of a clinical trial include

   a. development of a testable hypothesis
   b. development of a baseline state
   c. selection of interventions and comparisons
   d. all of the above

25–3. The use of placebos in clinical trials can be supported by which of the following?

   a. The treatment drug is clearly superior to placebo.
   b. Informed consent is required.
   c. The chances of the subject receiving the placebo are not important.
   d. none of the above

25–4. Which of the following is true with regard to randomization in clinical trials?

   a. It creates comparable study groups.
   b. Alternating assignments of subjects to a group is a form of randomization.
   c. The validity of statistical tests is not justified on the basis of randomization alone.
   d. all of the above

25–5. Cross-over trial designs include all of the following EXCEPT

   a. single and double designs
   b. reduced costs of a study
   c. requirement of a long washout
   d. the use of treatments that cure the condition

25–6. Which of the following is true regarding single-blind studies?

   a. Participants are blinded.
   b. Investigators are blinded.
   c. They can be used in comparison of surgical versus medical therapy.
   d. Initiating and maintaining them is difficult.

25–7. Adverse events in a clinical trial include all of the following EXCEPT

 a. they are usually well defined
 b. the investigator can elicit adverse events
 c. the events can be volunteered by the participants
 d. subject diaries require an enormous amount of time and cost to review

25–8. The components of a power analysis include

 a. budget
 b. blinding of the subjects
 c. randomization
 d. probability of a type II (β) error

25–9. A type II or β error includes which of the following?

 a. The investigator falsely rejects the null hypothesis.
 b. The investigator falsely accepts the null hypothesis.
 c. The investigator fails to find an outcome when one really exists.
 d. The investigator fails to randomize appropriately.

25–10. The β or type II error is often set at 0.20, which makes the power of the study

 a. 20 percent
 b. 0.2 percent
 c. 80 percent
 d. 95 percent

25–11. The type I (α) error is usually set at what percentage?

 a. 5 percent
 b. 20 percent
 c. 80 percent
 d. 95 percent

25–12. A phase I study includes which of the following?

 a. designed to determine drug efficacy
 b. comprises a large number of subjects
 c. studies rate of adverse events
 d. determines metabolic and pharmacologic action of a drug

25–13. The postmenopausal estrogen/progestin interventions (PEPI) hormone replacement trial is which of the following studies?

 a. phase I
 b. phase II
 c. phase III
 d. phase IV

25–14. Which of the following tests studies the association between two variables (ie, heart disease and high-density lipoprotein [HDL]) in which the sample size is small and nonparametric?

 a. Mantel–Haenszel statistic
 b. Student's t test
 c. Spearman's rank correlation
 d. Fisher's exact test

25–15. The method of calculation of the relative risk includes

 a. the Mantel–Haenszel method
 b. the random effect model
 c. the 95 percent confidence interval
 d. all of the above

25–16. Who was credited with introducing the principles of randomization to clinical trials?

 a. Fisher
 b. Johnson
 c. Jones
 d. Fishburn

25–17. Which of the following groups are required for clinical trials of new drugs by the U.S. Food and Drug Administration (FDA)?

 a. pregnant women
 b. children
 c. African Americans
 d. none of the above

25–18. Which of the following is a significant problem with infertility studies?

 a. lack of prospective trials
 b. insufficient power
 c. lack of placebo arms
 d. all of the above

25–19. The primary uses of clinical trials for the evaluation of pharmacologic agents include all of the following EXCEPT

   a. safety
   b. efficacy
   c. efficiency
   d. effectiveness

25–20. Which of the following is most appropriate to evaluate the effect of gonadotropins on the incidence of ovarian cancer?

   a. retrospective analysis
   b. case-controlled study
   c. prospective, randomized, placebo-controlled trial
   d. none of the above

25–21. Which of the following entrance criteria may be required in developing a clinical trial for the treatment of endometriosis?

   a. history of dysmenorrhea
   b. infertility
   c. biopsy-proven endometriosis
   d. all of the above

25–22. Which type of history should be a reason to exclude a patient from a study of medical treatment for endometriosis pain?

   a. previous pregnancy
   b. Crohn's disease
   c. family history of endometriosis
   d. previous use of contraceptives

25–23. All of the following describe most volunteers in clinical trials EXCEPT

   a. welfare recipients
   b. healthy patients
   c. Caucasians
   d. higher education

25–24. Randomized protocols can be

   a. equal
   b. proportional
   c. both of the above
   d. none of the above

25–25. Which of the following best describes the benefits in a randomization method by strata or blocks in a small study?

   a. will provide equal patients into a study
   b. helps to distribute evenly prognostic variables that are closely associated
   c. easy to recruit subjects
   d. all of the above

25–26. All of the following are principal criteria of study budget costs EXCEPT

   a. personnel
   b. equipment
   c. supplies
   d. advertising

25–27. A chi-square test is not appropriate if the expected frequency is less than

   a. 1 percent
   b. 5 percent
   c. 10 percent
   d. 15 percent

REPRODUCTIVE MEDICINE AND THE MANAGED CARE MARKET

26–1. Which of the following states has liberal mandated coverage for assisted reproductive technology?

    a. Massachusetts
    b. Maryland
    c. Illinois
    d. all of the above

26–2. Infertility affects which percentage of the population?

    a. 9 percent
    b. 11 percent
    c. 25 percent
    d. all of the above

26–3. Which of the following is true regarding medical service organizations?

    a. They are privately held entities.
    b. Ownership is generally split between physicians and hospitals.
    c. Recent relaxation of antitrust laws has allowed these organizations to flourish.
    d. all of the above

26–4. The fastest growing form of managed care in 1997 is

    a. individual practice association (IPA)
    b. preferred provider organization (PPO)
    c. managed service organization (MSO)
    d. physician practice management (PPM)

26–5. What is the principal disadvantage to the PPM service?

    a. The PPM is involved in contract negotiations.
    b. The PPM furnishes group purchasing power.
    c. The professional corporation is separated from the PPM.
    d. The PPM handles billing and collections.

26–6. The statement "The conscientious, explicit, and judicious use of current best evidence in making decisions about the care of individual patients" describes

    a. disease management
    b. evidence-based medicine
    c. cost-effective analysis
    d. meta-analysis

26–7. Which best describes reproduction after the age of 35?

    a. There is an exponential fall in fecundity rate.
    b. There is an exponential rise in the incidence of trisomies.
    c. There is an exponential rise in pregnancy loss.
    d. all of the above

26–8. Which of the following does NOT increase after the age of 35?

a. ectopic pregnancy
b. congenital malformation
c. placenta previa
d. none of the above

26–9. Algorithms used in reproductive medicine do which of the following?

a. codify the standard of practice
b. make therapy finite
c. control cost
d. all of the above

26–10. Infertility results in hidden cost to employers, including

a. depression of employees
b. marital discord
c. isolation of the couple
d. all of the above

26–11. Which of the following is NOT a pitfall encountered in managed care contracting?

a. retroactive payment denial
b. indemnification clauses
c. termination at will
d. all of the above

26–12. From the point of view of economics, clomiphene citrate produces its most efficient result after what time period?

a. 3 months
b. 5 months
c. 8 months
d. 12 months

26–13. Which of the following is associated with a systematic approach to evaluate the outcomes and costs of intervention?

a. evidence-based medicine
b. disease management
c. Delphi analysis
d. cost-effective analysis

26–14. Which of the following is NOT a PPM service?

a. MedPartners
b. HealthSouth
c. Principal Care
d. Gyncor

26–15. All of the following have been cited as current problems in U.S. health care EXCEPT

a. oversupply of U.S.-trained physicians
b. influx of foreign medical practitioners
c. utilization of high-tech services
d. all of the above

26–16. Which of the following institutions was credited with devising the contemporary case report?

a. Johns Hopkins
b. Harvard Medical School
c. New York Hospital
d. Mayo Clinic

26–17. Which of the following has contributed to unfavorable public opinion regarding infertility treatment?

a. lack of public education
b. sensationalism by contemporary news magazines
c. behavior by infertility practitioners
d. all of the above

26–18. Which of the following individuals released a report in 1910 evaluating medical education in the United States and Canada?

a. Abraham Flexner
b. John Shaw Billings
c. Daniel Coit Gilman
d. William Henry Welch

26–19. Which of the following individuals was named to the first chair of gynecology at Johns Hopkins University?

a. William Henry Welch
b. William Mosler
c. William Stuart Halsted
d. Howard Atwood Kelly

26–20. Which of the following individuals pioneered bladder fistula surgery and established a major women's hospital in New York?

    a. Hunter Robb
    b. W.T.G. Morton
    c. Crawford W. Long
    d. J. Marion Sims

26–21. Which of the following individuals was not a partner in the original Mayo Clinic?

    a. Henry S. Plummer
    b. Edward Starr Judd
    c. Marvin Millett
    d. Ephram McDowell

26–22. In which of the following years was Louise Brown born in Oldham General District Hospital in Lancaster, England?

    a. 1975
    b. 1978
    c. 1980
    d. 1982

26–23. Data from the national registry suggest that what percentage of patients never seek infertility care?

    a. 10 percent
    b. 25 percent

    c. 43 percent
    d. 50 percent

26–24. Data from large HMOs show that what percentage of patients who are infertile seek treatment in a given year?

    a. 5 percent
    b. 10 to 12 percent
    c. 25 percent
    d. 50 percent

26–25. Which of the following is associated with an oversupply of U.S. physicians?

    a. the production of 17,000 U.S. graduates per year
    b. maldistribution of specialists
    c. inflow of 8000 foreign medical practitioners per year
    d. all of the above

26–26. Which of the following will help physicians regain control of the health care market?

    a. reduction of residency and fellowship training slots
    b. acquisition of business and legal skills by physicians
    c. use of evidence-based medicine and cost-effective analysis
    d. all of the above

Chapter 27

DIAGNOSTIC EVALUATION AND TREATMENT ALGORITHMS FOR THE INFERTILE COUPLE

CASE REPORT

The patient is a 31-year-old white female, para 0-0-2-0, with ectopic pregnancies in 1993 and 1997, both of which occurred in the right fallopian tube. She had undergone two salpingostomies; however, hysterosalpingogram (HSG) performed after her last surgery showed occlusion of the right fallopian tube distally. The left fallopian tube demonstrated prompt spill and fill, and the uterine cavity was normal.

The patient underwent menarche at age 13, denied a history of galactorrhea, and had irregular menstrual cycles ranging from 25 to 40 days. She denied a history of dysmenorrhea or dyspareunia.

Her infertility workup consisted of a semen analysis which showed a volume of 3 cc, count of 100 million sperm/cc, 60 percent motility, and 80 percent normal morphology. In view of her cycle irregularity, she had been treated with clomiphene citrate for 1 month at a dose of 50 mg/day on cycle days 3 through 7. A postcoital test was carried out during that cycle, and one timed to a luteinizing hormone (LH) surge kit showed thick mucus with sperm present demonstrating minimum motility. The patient experienced a number of side effects during clomiphene treatment including mood lability, headache, and lethargy. She was not interested in taking further cycles of clomiphene citrate.

Her past medical history was unremarkable with the exception of two ectopic surgeries. Her social history revealed a professional background. The patient drank a moderate amount of alcohol socially; had a 10-year history of smoking, which she had discontinued several months earlier; and had a history of recreational drug use in college.

Physical examination showed a height of 5'6", weight 132 lb, and normal vital signs. No thyromegaly was detected, nor was galactorrhea. The patient had no signs of hirsutism, and her examination was normal with the exception of two suprapubic and one umbilical scar secondary to laparoscopy.

In view of her ovulatory irregularity, the patient was evaluated for hypothyroidism and hyperprolactinemia. She was found to be euthyroid and euprolactinemic, suggesting a hypothalamic origin of her ovulatory dysfunction. The patient was presented with two therapeutic options: a limited trial of superovulation with urofollitropin (Fertinex) plus intrauterine insemination, or in vitro fertilization. She and her husband elected the former therapy.

SUMMARY AND CONCLUSIONS

Ectopic pregnancy occurs in approximately 1 in 200 pregnancies in the population at large. Risk factors include ovulatory dysfunction, endometriosis, pelvic infection and/or previous tubal surgery, and possibly exposure to diethylstilbestrol in utero. While this patient's risk of recurrent ectopic pregnancy is significant, financial constraints often make the use of assisted reproductive technology prohibitive.

Gonadotropins, while originally developed for the induction of ovulation, have been utilized in a variety of infertility strategies including improvement of folliculogenesis, improvement of cervical mucus, induction of superovulation, or manipulation at the site of ovulation in cases of impaired tubal function. In the latter case, this strategy allows ovulation to consistently occur near a patent fallopian tube.

This case also brings to light another important issue, that is, delay in ovulation. It was shown many years ago by Louis Rodriguez-Rigau that women who ovulate later than day 16 have a markedly reduced fecundity rate. At least two mechanisms are involved in this reduction in fertility: (1) luteinization without ovulation, and (2) the ovulation of immature oocytes. Care must be taken to separate luteinization from ovulation. This could best be done by the utilization of sequential sonography combined with the urinary measurement of an LH surge. Often, clusters of small follicles will be found, each producing a small but significant amount of estrogen that induces a blunted LH surge. If enough follicle-stimulating hormone (FSH) has been present to induce LH receptors on granulosa cells, luteinization will occur, often yielding normal progesterone levels. On the other hand, delayed folliculogenesis will often generate enough estrogen feedback to induce minispikes of LH. While not inducing ovulation, it may bring about the resumption of meiosis. This gives rise to the ovulation some time later of an immature follicle. The latter condition is diagnosed by the presence of a mature follicle at midcycle, yet delay of 4 to 5 days in the LH surge. Both of these conditions can often be managed with clomiphene administration with or without timed human chorionic gonadotropin (hCG) injection or the use of FSH therapy.

BIBLIOGRAPHY

Prough SE, Axsel S, Yowman R. Luteinizing hormone: bioactivity invariable responses to clomiphene citrate and chronic anovulation. *Fertil Steril.* 54:799, 1990

Rodriguez-Rigau LJ, Shenoi PN, Smith KD, et al. The relationship between the links of the follicular and luteal phases of the menstrual cycle and the fertility potential of the female. *Fertil Steril.* 39:856, 1983

Ying YK, Daly DC, Randolph JF, et al. Ultrasonographic monitoring of follicle growth for luteal phase defect. *Fertil Steril.* 48:433, 1987

QUESTIONS

27–1. What percentage of women age 35 to 39 will conceive within 1 year of unprotected intercourse?

  a. 50 percent
  b. 75 percent
  c. 85 percent
  d. 90 percent

27–2. What percentage of the causes of infertility in a couple are due to male factors?

  a. 15 percent
  b. 25 percent
  c. 35 percent
  d. 55 percent

27–3. Cigarette smoking may be associated with

  a. late menopause
  b. increased sperm motility
  c. increased libido
  d. delayed time for conception

27–4. A 22-year-old female presents with infertility for 1 year. Which tests should be included in the initial evaluation?

  a. postcoital
  b. serum FSH
  c. hysterosalpingogram (HSG)
  d. sonohysterography

27–5. The usefulness of the basal body temperature (BBT) includes all of the following EXCEPT

  a. accurately predicting day of ovulation
  b. confirming a short luteal phase
  c. confirming an ovulatory cycle
  d. a temperature rise of 0.4 °F is characteristic of luteal phase

27–6. An endometrial biopsy for infertility is associated with all of the following EXCEPT

    a. a 3-day delay in maturation confirms a short luteal phase

    b. it is obtained from the anterior wall of the fundus

    c. it can be correlated with LH surge

    d. it is performed 1 to 2 days prior to menses

27–7. At what age in infertile women has it been suggested to screen with a day 3 FSH level?

    a. 30

    b. 33

    c. 35

    d. 40

27–8. Which of the following instruments provides the best results in performing an HSG?

    a. pediatric Foley catheter

    b. HUI (balloon catheter)

    c. Jarco cannula

    d. NOVY catheter

27–9. How much radiopaque dye will usually fill the uterine cavity during an HSG?

    a. 2 cc

    b. 5 cc

    c. 8 cc

    d. 15 cc

27–10. Which days of the cycle are ideal for performing an HSG?

    a. 3 to 5

    b. 5 to 7

    c. 7 to 11

    d. 11 to 13

27–11. All of the following are related to the role of laparoscopy in the infertile woman EXCEPT it

    a. is best performed in early to mid-follicular phase

    b. is indicated if an HSG suggests tubal occlusion

    c. is best performed at time of ovulation for confirmation of follicular rupture

    d. may identify abnormality in 20 percent of women

27–12. Which of the following is true regarding the postcoital test?

    a. It is a good predictor of cervical pathology.

    b. It can be performed anytime during the follicular phase from day 7 to 14.

    c. No standardization of method is available.

    d. It is a good predictor of fertility.

27–13. At what point in the infertility evaluation is therapeutic psychological intervention encouraged?

    a. at initiation of therapy

    b. when depression is noted

    c. pregnancy loss

    d. all of the above

27–14. A 34-year-old female with 4 years of infertility and early history of polycystic ovary syndrome (PCOS) failed to ovulate on clomiphene citrate 50 to 150 mg for three cycles. All of the following are accepted treatments EXCEPT

    a. increasing to 200 mg clomiphene

    b. monitoring follicular growth with ultrasound

    c. adding progesterone suppositories

    d. administering low-dose gonadotropins

27–15. In a 32-year-old female with 1 year of unexplained infertility, what is the first appropriate treatment?

    a. clomiphene citrate

    b. clomiphene citrate plus intrauterine insemination

    c. menotropins

    d. menotropins plus intrauterine insemination

27–16. All of the following may be appropriate in the treatment or evaluation of an infertile couple with a severe male factor EXCEPT

    a. intrauterine insemination
    b. referral to a urologist
    c. in vitro fertilization (IVF) with intracytoplasmic sperm injection (ICSI)
    d. donor sperm

27–17. Which of the following is NOT indicated if a questionable abnormal filling defect is reported on an HSG?

    a. assuming it is not significant
    b. evaluating the HSG film
    c. office hysteroscopy
    d. sonohysterography

27–18. Which of the following is most likely to be true in a woman with infertility at age 40?

    a. The risk of abortion is equal to that of a 30-year-old woman.
    b. A day 3 FSH test is indicated.
    c. The evaluation of a male should include a sperm penetration assay.
    d. all of the above

27–19. Evaluation or treatment of a unilateral proximal occlusion on HSG includes

    a. repeating the HSG immediately
    b. office hysteroscopy
    c. laparotomy with tubal implantation
    d. laparoscopy with hysteroscopy-directed tubal cannulation

27–20. The initial treatment of a young couple with 3 years of unexplained infertility includes

    a. laparoscopy
    b. gamete intrafallopian transfer (GIFT)
    c. clomiphene citrate plus intrauterine insemination
    d. none of the above

27–21. Which of the following best describes the postcoital test?

    a. Established criteria are available.
    b. It correlates well with sperm penetration assay.
    c. It correlates well with sperm motility.
    d. It correlates well with immunobead testing.

27–22. Which day of the cycle is a serum progesterone test obtained?

    a. any day
    b. day 14
    c. day 26
    d. none of the above

27–23. A triple line seen on ultrasonography indicates

    a. low estrogen
    b. high progesterone
    c. high estrogen
    d. low FSH

27–24. A problem that can occur during or following an HSG is

    a. infection
    b. pain
    c. allergic reaction
    d. all of the above

27–25. Which of the following is indicated in a couple with mild oligospermia on an initial semen analysis?

    a. referral to a urologist
    b. avoiding frequent intercourse
    c. donor sperm
    d. none of the above

27–26. Laparoscopy should be performed during an infertility evaluation

    a. in all couples
    b. in all cases in which distal tubal occlusion is seen on HSG
    c. on day 15 of the cycle
    d. none of the above

27–27. Which of the following is NOT an appropriate early choice in cases of mild distal tubal disease at laparoscopy?

    a. in vitro fertilization and embryo transfer (IVF-ET)
    b. surgery followed with clomiphene plus intrauterine insemination (IUI)
    c. surgery followed by IUI
    d. surgery followed by observation

Chapter 28

DIAGNOSIS AND TREATMENT OF MALE INFERTILITY

CASE REPORT

A 24-year-old male with a 2-year history of infertility was found to have an abnormal semen analysis (Table 28–1). The test was repeated and confirmed the initial result. He had a history of insulin-dependent diabetes mellitus for 6 years and was currently well controlled. The physical exam revealed a normal, well-developed male, 6′3″, 190 lb, with normal male phenotype, normal axillary and pubic hair, and normal male genitalia. The testes were of normal size. The vas deferens was palpable.

Additional laboratory tests revealed a follicle-stimulating hormone (FSH) level of 4 mIU/ml, a luteinizing hormone (LH) level of 6 mIU/ml, and a testosterone level of 7 ng/ml.

A urine analysis was obtained soon after ejaculation, which revealed numerous motile sperm. The diagnosis of retrograde ejaculation was made.

Prior to treatment, an evaluation of his spouse's fertility included a normal hysterosalpingogram (HSG) and day 21 progesterone. She began testing urine for an LH surge and on day 12 noted ovulation. The husband was taking $NaHCO_3$ (sodium bicarbonate), 300 mg, every day beginning on day 11. After masturbation, he voided and the urine sample was washed with Baker's solution and centrifuged for 10 minutes at 1500 rpm. The supernatant was discarded and the sperm pellet resuspended in Baker's solution (1 to 2 ml), and his wife was inseminated on day 13. She conceived and delivered a term infant.

SUMMARY AND CONCLUSIONS

Azoospermia should be confirmed on at least two semen analyses subjected to centrifugation. If the hormonal analyses are normal, then the subsequent evaluation depends on the presence of fructose in the ejaculate. In the presence of a palpable vas (which sometimes requires sonography or magnetic resonance imaging [MRI]), the postejaculatory urine will confirm retrograde ejaculation. Retrograde ejaculations are due to autonomic neuropathy, most commonly due to diabetes or a complication of surgery. Treatment includes an α-sympathomimetic drug (ephedrine), oral alkalinization, or instillation of an alkaline solution directly into the bladder followed by timed intrauterine insemination (IUI).

Table 28–1. Semen Analysis of Subject

Volume	0.5 ml
Color	Cloudy
Count	0×10^6
Motility	ND
Morphology	ND
Fructose	Negative
Diagnosis	Azoospermia

ND = Not Determined.

BIBLIOGRAPHY

MacLeod J. Human male infertility. *Obstet Gynecol Surv.* 26:325, 1971

McConnell JD. Diagnosis and treatment of male infertility. In: Carr BR, Blackwell RE, eds. *Textbook of Reproductive Medicine*, 1st ed. Norwalk, CT, Appleton & Lange, 1993: 453–468

Sigman M, Lipshultz LI, Howards SS. Evaluation of the sub-
fertile male. In: Marshall D, ed. *Infertility in the Male.* St.
Louis, MO, Mosby-Year Book, 1985: 179–210

Simmons FA. Human infertility. *N Engl J Med.* 225:110, 1956

QUESTIONS

28–1. In what percentage of couples with infertility are both male and female factors found?

    a. 10 percent
    b. 20 percent
    c. 30 percent
    d. 40 percent

28–2. Which of the following is NOT appropriate if, during the initial evaluation of the infertile couple, azoospermia is found on the first sample?

    a. Repeat the test.
    b. Examine the male.
    c. Halt the workup of the female until the etiology is discovered.
    d. Take a history from the male partner.

28–3. What percentage of postpubertal males who develop mumps parotitis develop orchitis?

    a. 25 percent
    b. 50 percent
    c. 75 percent
    d. 100 percent

28–4. What is the volume of a normal adult testis using an orchidometer?

    a. 5 ml
    b. 10 ml
    c. 15 ml
    d. 25 ml

28–5. Which of the following is true regarding a varicocele?

    a. The majority occur on the left side.
    b. The size of the varicocele does not correlate with the semen analysis.
    c. Venography has not improved pregnancy rates.
    d. all of the above

28–6. Which of the following is NOT acceptable with regard to the semen analysis?

    a. There should be an abstinence period of ≥ 7 days.
    b. Two or three analyses may be required.
    c. Fructose should be measured if volume is 1 ml or less.
    d. Motility should be promptly assessed.

28–7. All of the following are characteristic of a normal semen analysis (minimum standards) EXCEPT

    a. volume of 1.5 to 5.0 cc
    b. motility >40 percent
    c. forward progression >2
    d. morphology (strict) >15 percent

28–8. In a male with oligospermia less than 10×10^6/ml, which of the following tests is least useful?

    a. prolactin
    b. LH
    c. testosterone
    d. FSH

28–9. Which of the following tests confirms the presence of immunoglobulin A (IgA) antibodies attached to the tail of the sperm?

    a. agglutination tests
    b. hypo-osmotic testing
    c. immunobead test
    d. sperm penetration assay (SPA)

28–10. What percentage of normal, fertile males will test negatively on the SPA?

    a. 5 percent
    b. 10 percent
    c. 15 percent
    d. 20 percent

28–11. Which of the following is NOT associated or characterized by the computer-assisted motion analysis?

    a. accurate measurement of sperm velocity
    b. detection of sperm linearity
    c. expensive equipment
    d. predicts infertility better than standard semen analysis

28–12. A testicular biopsy should be performed in which of the following circumstances?

a. oligospermia
b. azoospermic males with high FSH
c. small testes with high FSH
d. none of the above

28–13. If a male presents with azoospermia with absence of fructose in the seminal fluid but normal plasma testosterone, what is the diagnosis?

a. ejaculatory duct obstruction
b. retrograde ejaculation
c. agenesis of vas deferens
d. all of the above

28–14. Treatment of antisperm antibodies resulting in increased pregnancy rates includes

a. dexamethasone
b. prednisone
c. plasmapheresis
d. none of the above

28–15. Which of the following therapies for male infertility has been proven effective?

a. testosterone
b. empiric thyroid
c. testolactone
d. none of the above

28–16. In what percentage of infertile couples is there a significant male factor present?

a. 10 percent
b. 20 percent
c. 30 percent
d. 50 percent

28–17. What is considered the minimal acceptable sperm count on semen analysis ($\times 10^6$)?

a. 10
b. 20
c. 60
d. 100

28–18. All of the following can lead to ejaculatory dysfunction (ie, retrograde ejaculation) EXCEPT

a. multiple sclerosis
b. genital surgery
c. tuberculosis
d. diabetes mellitus

28–19. What is the effect of anabolic steroids on semen quality?

a. slight increase
b. significant increase
c. decrease
d. no effect

28–20. If a male developed a severe febrile illness on January 1 that lasted 10 days, what would be the semen analysis quality on February 1?

a. no change
b. decrease
c. slight increase
d. decreased count, increased motility

28–21. Which of the following syndromes describes a man with chronic sinopulmonary disease, situs inversus, and nonmotile sperm?

a. Kallmann
b. Krukenberg
c. Kaperstein
d. none of the above

28–22. Which of the following has been clearly proven to impair spermatogenesis?

a. hot tub
b. sauna
c. steam bath
d. none of the above

28–23. Which of the following is an essential indication to obtain a hormone analysis in infertile men?

a. azoospermia
b. normal count, decreased motility
c. abnormal morphology
d. all of the above

28–24. All of the following are clearly associated with the development of antisperm antibodies EXCEPT

    a. vasectomy
    b. testicular torsion
    c. testicular biopsy
    d. genital duct obstruction

28–25. Round cells seen on the semen analysis are caused by

    a. excessive exercise
    b. marijuana
    c. infection
    d. all of the above

28–26. Which of the following is an indication for vasography?

    a. azoospermia
    b. azoospermia with biopsy-proven spermatogenesis
    c. oligospermia
    d. all of the above

28–27. What is the fructose content in men with retrograde ejaculation?

    a. reduced 25 percent
    b. reduced 50 percent
    c. reduced 75 percent
    d. reduced 100 percent

Chapter 29

OVULATION INDUCTION

CASE REPORT

The patient is a 27-year-old white female, para 0-0-0-0, who presents with a lifelong history of irregular menstruation. She denies any galactorrhea, increased body hair growth, acne, or oily skin. Likewise, she denies dry skin, cold intolerance, or constipation. She also denies any increase or decrease in body weight. She went through puberty and started menstruation at 11 years of age. She gave a history of having been treated with oral contraceptive agents since the late teens for cycle regulation, and, as expected, her irregular menstruation returned after discontinuing the birth control pills.

Physical examination showed a well-nourished female, height 5′5″, and weight 128 lb. No thyromegaly was palpated. She had no evidence of hyperandrogenemia, no discharge could be expressed from the breasts, and the remainder of her physical examination including pelvic exam was normal.

The following endocrine profile was obtained: luteinizing hormone (LH), 7 mIU/ml; follicle-stimulating hormone (FSH), 4 mIU/ml; prolactin (PRL), 10 ng/ml; and high-sensitivity thyroid-stimulating hormone (TSH), 4 mIU/ml.

The initial impression was that this patient had chronic hypothalamic anovulation. A urine pregnancy test was found to be negative, and she was given 100 mg of progesterone in oil intramuscularly (IM). This produced menstruation 5 days later, and she was started on clomiphene citrate, 50 mg/day, on days 2 through 6. Monitoring consisted of basal body temperature (BBT) chart analysis, the use of urinary ovulation predictor kits on days 11 through 16, and mid-luteal progesterone determination on days 22 and 23. The patient failed to demonstrate any evidence of ovulation on clomiphene doses of 50, 100, 150, and 200 mg/day. Sonography obtained on day 15 in the absence of a urinary LH surge showed multiple small follicles, apparently 1.1 cm in size.

In view of the poor response to clomiphene, the patient was started on gonadotropin therapy and was treated with Pergonal for three cycles, each of which produced adequate evidence of ovulation as determined by multiple sonograms and estrogen determinations. On the fourth cycle, she received 30 ampules of gonadotropin over a 10-day period and had an estradiol level of 1432 pg/ml on the day of human chorionic gonadotropin (hCG) administration. She had three mature follicles—1.9, 1.7, and 1.6 cm—distributed between both ovaries, yet had 4 to 5 other follicles, which were 1.4 cm in size.

Eight days after administration of 10,000 units of hCG, the patient began to develop abdominal distention and pain. Sonogram showed that the ovaries were approximately 6 cm in size (Fig. 29–1). The patient had no nausea or vomiting; however, over the next 3 days, she experienced an increase in abdominal girth, pain, and body weight. Her hematocrit had become concentrated from 37 to 47 percent, and she complained of persistent nausea and dyspnea. The ovaries scanned at over 10 cm in size, and ascites was noted to be present.

She was admitted to the hospital for hydration and pain control. A Foley catheter was placed and D5-1/2 normal saline was administered at a rate to maintain urine output at between 20 and 30 cc/hr. Chest x-ray was normal, as were blood gases; however, after 5 days of hospitalization she had gained a total of 30 lb above her pre-gonadotropin treatment weight. She had progressive dyspnea and un-

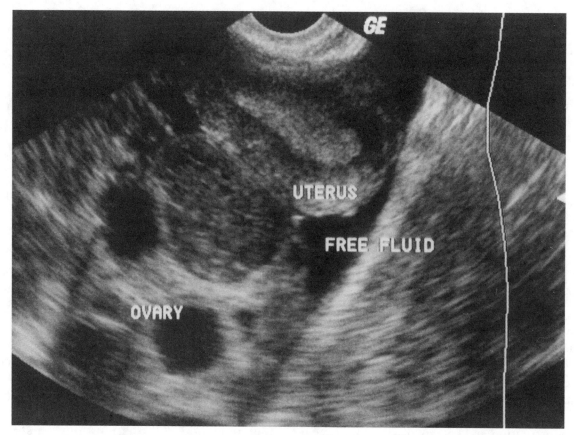

Figure 29–1. Transvaginal sonogram showing severe hyperstimulation in patient taking gonadotropins.

derwent paracentesis, at which time 1700 ml of acidic fluid was removed. Fortunately, she entered a state of diuresis 3 days later and was discharged from the hospital on day 17 with a twin gestation.

SUMMARY AND CONCLUSIONS

This patient represents a classic pattern as seen in the individual with severe ovarian hyperstimulation syndrome. The condition invariably occurs following the administration of hCG and appears 7 to 8 days after the injection. If pregnancy does not occur, the problem usually resolves within about another 8 to 10 days. However, as fetal hCG begins to rise, particularly if multiple gestations are present, the ovaries receive added stimulation. Patients generally complain of weight gain, nausea, vomiting, increased abdominal girth, and pain. The hallmarks for admission of the patient with hyperstimulation syndrome includes a rising hematocrit, increased abdominal pain, or the inability to tolerate fluids orally. Once admitted to the hospital, the object of therapy is balanced hydration, prevention of hemoconcentration and subsequent emboli, and control of pain. The hospital course will be dictated by whether a multiple gestation is present.

BIBLIOGRAPHY

Paoletti AM, Cagnacci A, Depau GF, et al. The chronic administration of cabergoline normalizes androgen secretion and improves menstrual cyclicity in women with polycystic ovary syndrome. *Fertil Steril.* 66:527, 1996

Shoham Z, Insler V. Recombinant technique and gonadotropin production: new era in reproductive medicine. *Fertil Steril.* 66:187, 1996

Tan SL, Farhi J, Homburg R, Jacobs HS. Induction of ovulation in clomiphene-resistant polycystic ovary syndrome with pulsatile GnRH. *Obstet Gynecol.* 88:221, 1996

Trott EA, Plouffe L Jr, Hansen K, et al. Ovulation induction in clomiphene-resistant anovulatory women with normal dehydroepiandrosterone sulfate levels: beneficial effects of the addition of dexamethasone during the follicular phase. *Fertil Steril.* 66:484, 1996

Wilcox AJ, Weinberg CR, Baird DD. Timing of sexual intercourse in relation to ovulation. *N Engl J Med.* 333:1517, 1995

QUESTIONS

29-1. All of the following describe World Health Organization (WHO) group I patients EXCEPT

    a. they may have elevated prolactin levels

    b. their serum gonadotropin levels are lower than normal

    c. they show estradiol levels in the postmenopausal range

    d. they do not demonstrate withdrawal bleeding to progestogen administration

29-2. Conditions included in WHO group I are

    a. Kallmann syndrome

    b. anorexia nervosa

    c. isolated gonadotropin deficiency

    d. all of the above

29-3. Which of the following is NOT true regarding use of the BBT chart for ovulatory monitoring?

    a. The BBT is monophasic in 12 to 20 percent of cycles.

    b. Temperature elevation usually occurs between days 11 and 16 in a normal ovulatory cycle.

    c. The BBT can be used to accurately predict oocyte release.

    d. A gradual temperature rise may indicate ovulatory dysfunction.

29-4. Which of the following is true regarding the LH surge?

    a. Ovulation occurs 20 hours after the onset of the LH surge.

    b. The midcycle rise in FSH tends to occur before LH.

    c. There is a lag time of 10 hours between serum and urinary LH surges.

    d. The LH surge usually begins between 5 and 9 AM.

29-5. Which of the following statements is true regarding progesterone secretion?

    a. Progesterone levels ≥3 ng/ml are associated with the presence of secretory endometrium.

    b. Serum progesterone levels ≥8.8 ng/ml are found in 98 percent of spontaneous conception cycles.

    c. Follicle rupture is important for efficient progesterone production by the corpus luteum.

    d. all of the above

29-6. Which of the following is NOT true regarding the endometrial biopsy?

    a. Twenty percent of samples taken during conception cycles are abnormal.

    b. The incidence of abnormal biopsies is the same in women with proven fertility and in infertile patients.

    c. A single endometrial biopsy is adequate to determine a luteal-phase defect.

    d. The optimal time for an endometrial biopsy is thought to be 2 to 3 days prior to menstruation.

29-7. Which of the following is indicative of normal folliculogenesis at the time of ovulation?

    a. an endometrial thickness of 1.0 cm

    b. a mean follicle diameter between 1.6 and 2.2 cm

    c. a serum estradiol level of 250 to 300 pg/ml

    d. all of the above

29-8. Which of the following measurements is the best predictor of premature ovarian failure?

    a. cycle day 3 FSH level

    b. cycle day 3 LH level

    c. cycle day 3 LH/FSH ratio

    d. cycle day 3 estradiol level

29-9. Which of the following is the best predictor of late-onset adrenal hyperplasia?

    a. serum dehydroepiandrosterone sulfate (DHEAS) level

    b. serum total testosterone level

    c. serum 17-hydroxyprogesterone level drawn in the follicular phase

    d. sex hormone-binding globulin (SHBG) level

29–10. Which of the following ovulation-inducing agents might produce successful results in patients with WHO group I ovulatory dysfunction?

    a. pulsatile gonadotropin-releasing hormone (GnRH) administered intravenously

    b. daily injections of human menopausal gonadotropin (hMG)

    c. preparations of urofolicotropin

    d. all of the above

29–11. When using gonadotropin therapy, twin gestations frequently occur above which level?

    a. 500 pg/ml

    b. 1000 pg/ml

    c. 800 pg/ml

    d. 100 pg/ml

29–12. Which of the following statements is NOT true regarding ovulation induction in WHO group II patients?

    a. There is no difference in ovulation rate if clomiphene is begun on cycle days 2, 3, 4, or 5.

    b. Patients with DHEAS levels greater than 2800 ng/ml often respond to dexamethasone administration.

    c. The administration of leuprolide acetate to this group of patients converts them to a WHO group I status.

    d. Wedge resection of the ovaries produces normalization of ovulatory function 70 percent of the time.

29–13. Which method is most effective in avoiding hyperstimulation syndrome in a patient with a large number of follicles seen on sonography and an abnormally elevated estradiol level?

    a. Selectively reduce the oocyte number with needle aspiration.

    b. Cancel the cycle.

    c. Administer 5000 units of hCG instead of 10,000.

    d. Administer a pulse of Lupron.

29–14. Which of the following is characteristic of severe hyperstimulation syndrome?

    a. ovaries greater than 10 cm

    b. ascites

    c. dehydration, nausea, and vomiting

    d. all of the above

29–15. Ovulatory dysfunction makes up what portion of the infertile population?

    a. 10 percent

    b. 20 percent

    c. 30 percent

    d. 40 percent

29–16. Which group of patients would be included in WHO group III?

    a. hyperthecosis

    b. Kallmann syndrome

    c. polycystic ovary syndrome

    d. resistant ovary syndrome

29–17. Which of the following is a physical finding associated with WHO group II amenorrhea?

    a. watery cervical mucus

    b. rugated vaginal mucosa

    c. will withdraw to progesterone bleeding 50 percent of the time

    d. all of the above

29–18. Which of the following hormones energize to induce the LH surge?

    a. estrogen and FSH

    b. estrogen and activin

    c. estrogen and progesterone

    d. progesterone and PRL

29–19. Which progesterone level has been shown to be associated with the achievement of pregnancy?

    a. 8.8 ng/ml

    b. 10 ng/ml

    c. 15 ng/ml

    d. all of the above

29–20. Although endometrial biopsies have been considered the gold standard of confirming ovulation, the technique has which of the following major disadvantages?

   a. It is expensive.
   b. It can be uncomfortable for the patient.
   c. It is subject to great interpretation error.
   d. It is time consuming.

29–21. Which size follicle is capable of producing a viable pregnancy?

   a. 14 mm
   b. 16 mm
   c. 18 mm
   d. all of the above

29–22. Sonographic evidence of dysfolliculogenesis has been demonstrated in what percentage of regularly menstruating women with no other cause of infertility?

   a. 20 percent
   b. 30 percent
   c. 40 percent
   d. 50 percent

29–23. Which level of 17-hydroxyprogesterone is diagnostic for late-onset congenital adrenal hyperplasia when measured in the follicular phase?

   a. 1 ng/ml
   b. 2 ng/ml
   c. 4 ng/ml
   d. 6 ng/ml

29–24. Ovulatory dysfunction begins to occur as body weight increases to

   a. 105 percent of ideal
   b. 110 percent of ideal
   c. 115 percent of ideal
   d. 120 percent of ideal

29–25. Using native GnRH to induce ovulation in WHO group I patients, pulses should be delivered at intervals of

   a. 20 to 30 minutes
   b. 30 to 45 minutes
   c. 60 to 120 minutes
   d. 120 to 180 minutes

29–26. Which of the following is true regarding the chemistry of contemporary gonadotropins?

   a. They are purified from urine.
   b. They contain protein contaminants.
   c. They contain equal portions of FSH and LH.
   d. all of the above

29–27. The pregnancy rate achieved with gonadotropin therapy in WHO group I patients is

   a. 10 percent per cycle
   b. 20 percent per cycle
   c. 25 to 30 percent per cycle
   d. 40 percent per cycle

29–28. Which of the following statements is true regarding the two sterioisomers of clomiphene citrate?

   a. Enclomiphene is more biologically active than zuclomiphene.
   b. Enclomiphene is cleared from the body more rapidly than zuclomiphene.
   c. Zuclomiphene has greater potency than enclomiphene.
   d. Zuclomiphene is retained in the body lower than enclomiphene

Chapter 30

DIAGNOSIS AND TREATMENT OF UTERINE PATHOLOGY

CASE REPORT

A 14-year-old nulligravid patient was referred to the reproductive endocrinology clinic for evaluation of a vaginal mass (initially diagnosed as a Gartner's duct cyst) that had increased in size in the previous 2 years, accompanied by increasing dysmenorrhea. She denied any urinary or gastrointestinal complaints. She was sexually active and also had a re-

current vaginal discharge. Her pubertal development included breast development followed by menarche, which occurred at 11 to 12 years of age.

The physical exam revealed lower abdominal tenderness and a suggestion of a mass. The breasts were Tanner stage III, and the pelvic exam revealed normal external genitalia and pubic hair at Tanner stage III. A bulging cystic mass was identified originating from the left vaginal wall, filling the vagina and displacing the cervix upward. The vagi-

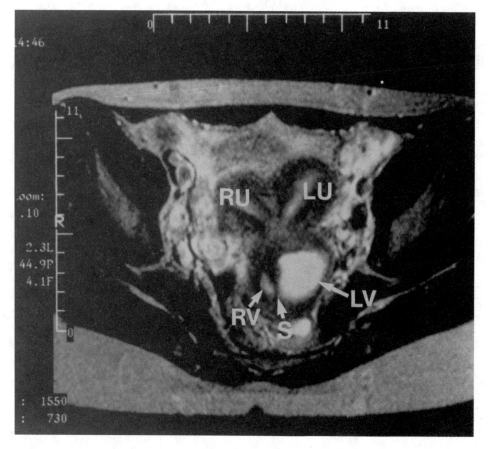

Figure 30–1. A cross-sectional (transverse section) MRI revealing both uteri (RU, LU), a small right vagina (RV), and large distended left vagina (LV). S, septum. *(Courtesy of Dr. Khaled Zeitoun, University of Texas Southwestern Medical Center at Dallas, Dallas, TX.)*

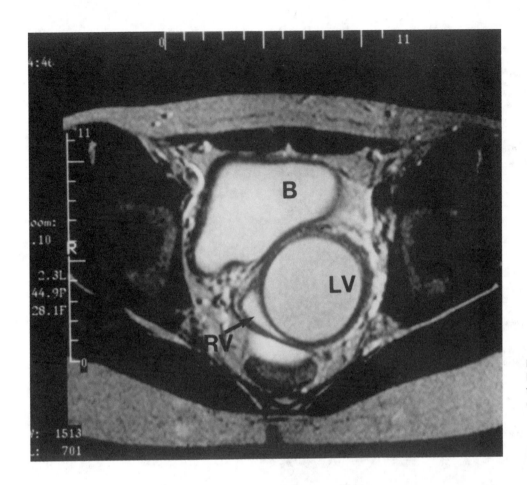

Figure 30–2. A cross-sectional MRI revealing the association of the bladder (B) with the left vagina (LV) and right vagina (RV). *(Courtesy of Dr. Khaled Zeitoun, University of Texas Southwestern Medical Center at Dallas, Dallas, TX.)*

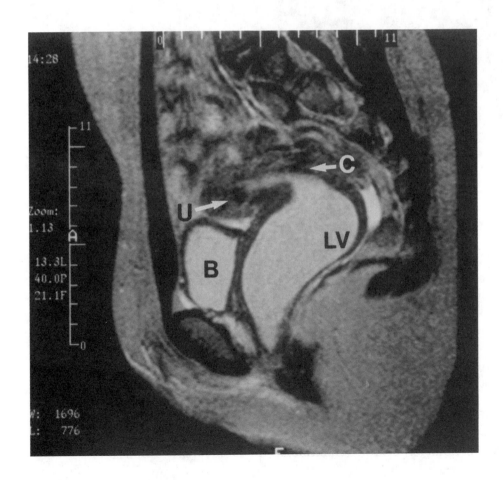

Figure 30–3. Longitudinal MRI revealing the bladder (B), left uterus (LU), and cervix (C), and the communication with the left vagina (LV). *(Courtesy of Dr. Khaled Zeitoun, University of Texas Southwestern Medical Center at Dallas, Dallas, TX.)*

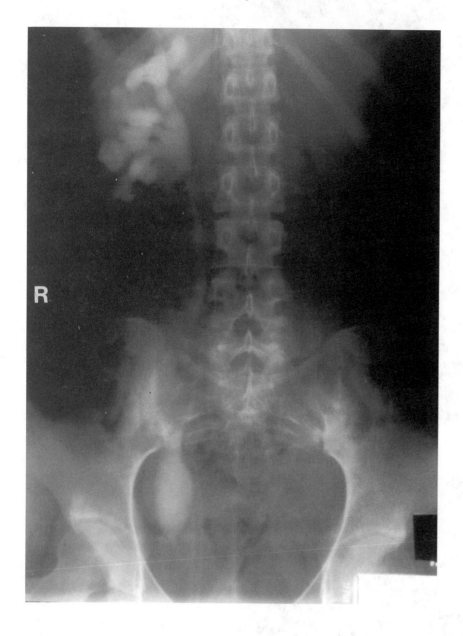

Figure 30–4. An intravenous pyelogram (IVP) demonstrating absence of the left kidney and ureter. *(Courtesy of Dr. Khaled Zeitoun, University of Texas Southwestern Medical Center at Dallas, Dallas, TX.)*

nal mass was felt continuous with the lower abdominal mass.

A magnetic resonance imaging (MRI) was performed, which revealed a double uterus, two cervices, and two vaginas. A hematometra was noted in the left uterus, and there was fluid (blood) in the right uterine cavity (due to communication between both uteri at the level of the internal os). In addition, a left obstructed hemivagina with large hematocolpos was observed (Figs 30–1 through 30–3). Finally, the left kidney was noted to be absent (Fig 30–4).

The patient underwent laparoscopy, which showed a duplicated uterus (uterus didelphys) with a distended left uterus (Fig 30–5). Both left and right uteri were fused in the midline at the level of the internal os. In addition, mild endometriosis of the peritoneum was seen, but the tubes and ovaries were normal. A wide excision of the vaginal septum was also performed, with drainage of red-tinged purulent material. A communication between both hemiuteri was confirmed. Two separate vaginas, cervices, and uteri were confirmed. The presence of this communication explains the infection noted and also the presence of only mild endometriosis and no hematosalpinx. The patient was treated with antibiotics, and her postoperative course was uncomplicated. Two weeks later, a follow-up examination revealed a normal vagina with two cervices identified.

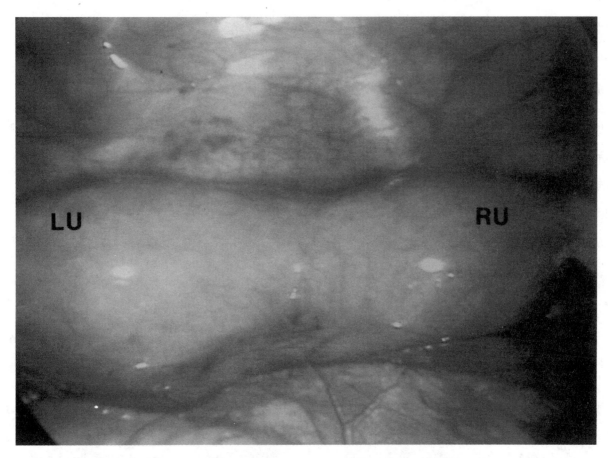

Figure 30–5. Laparoscopic view of the uterus didelphys with left (LU) and right (RU) uteri. *(Courtesy of Dr. Khaled Zeitoun, University of Texas Southwestern Medical Center at Dallas, Dallas, TX.)*

SUMMARY AND CONCLUSIONS

The double uterus, blind hemivagina, and ipsilateral renal agenesis complex is a rare malformation of the female urogenital system. The etiology of this malformation is thought to be primarily due to a defect in formation of the mesonephric duct. The mesonephric duct, which forms earlier than the Müllerian duct, is important for guiding the Müllerian ducts to the urogenital sinus. An interruption of the mesonephric duct will lead to defects in Müllerian duct formation as well as renal agenesis.

The clinical presentations of this disorder include: (1) dysmenorrhea that begins shortly after menarche and increases in severity with subsequent periods, (2) pelvic abdominal mass due to formation of a hematocolpos/hematometra and hematosalpinx, (3) endometriosis due to retrograde menstruation as seen in our case, and (4) vaginal discharge of a purulent nature in the presence of a communication between the obstructed hemiuterus or the hemivagina and the opposite side

where no obstruction is detected. In our case, we noted a communication between both uteri. A fistulous communication between the genital and urinary tracts has also been reported.

Diagnosis is best confirmed by an MRI or by ultrasonography. Prior to the use of modern imaging techniques, exploratory surgery often led to inadvertent hemihysterectomy, salpingectomy, or hemivaginectomy to remove a pelvic mass distended with menstrual blood.

Important additional points of this disorder include the following:

1. The association of unilateral renal agenesis (reported in almost all cases) with a pelvic mass is very suggestive of a Müllerian anomaly and should be kept in mind when cases of acute abdomen are encountered.
2. Treatment is by wide excision of the vaginal septum (simple incision or inadequate excision is associated with recurrence of the obstruction) and drainage of the collected menstrual blood.

Concomitant laparoscopy allows detection of the uterine anomaly and presence of associated endometriosis, which is reported to regress spontaneously after treatment.

3. Chances for subsequent fertility are good, and in approximately 75 percent of women, pregnancy has been reported after drainage of a large distended hematometra on the affected side. Thus, a hemihysterectomy or hysterectomy is rarely indicated in women desiring future fertility.

BIBLIOGRAPHY

Candiani GB, Fedele L, Candiani M. Double uterus, blind hemivagina, and ipsilateral renal agenesis: 36 cases and long-term follow-up. *Obstet Gynecol.* 90:26, 1997

Morgan MA, Thurnau GR, Smith ML. Uterus didelphys with unilateral hematocolpos, ipsilateral renal agenesis and menses. *J Reprod Med.* 32:47, 1987

Rock JA, Jones HW Jr. The double uterus associated with an obstructed hemivagina and ipsilateral renal agenesis. *Am J Obstet Gynecol.* 138:339, 1980

Shibata T, Nonomura K, Kakizaki H, et al. A case of unique communication between blind-ending ectopic ureter and ipsilateral hemi-hematocolpometra in uterus didelphys. *J Urol.* 153:1208, 1995

Stassart JP, Nagel TC, Prem KA, Phipps WR. Uterus didelphys, obstructed hemivagina, and ipsilateral renal agenesis: the University of Minnesota experience. *Fertil Steril.* 57:756, 1992

QUESTIONS

30–1. At which of the following weeks of fetal life do the Müllerian ducts form?

    a. 3 to 4
    b. 5 to 6
    c. 7 to 8
    d. 9 to 10

30–2. Which of the following defects in uterine development is associated with the highest incidence of reproductive loss?

    a. diethylstilbestrol (DES) anomaly
    b. uterus didelphys
    c. bicornuate uterus
    d. septate uterus

30–3. The hysterosalpingogram (HSG) is useful to diagnose which of the following uterine defects?

    a. uterine synechiae
    b. septate uterus
    c. bicornuate uterus
    d. all of the above

30–4. The Strassman surgical technique is the appropriate procedure for

    a. arcuate uterus
    b. septate uterus
    c. bicornuate uterus
    d. Rokitansky syndrome

30–5. Which of the following is NOT true regarding leiomyoma?

    a. There is an increase in size during pregnancy.
    b. Estrogen plasma levels are higher than normal.
    c. Estrogen receptor content is increased.
    d. Growth factors play a role in growth.

30–6. Which of the following have been reported to cause repeat pregnancy loss?

    a. pedunculated leiomyomas
    b. submucous leiomyomas
    c. multiple small serosal leiomyomas
    d. all of the above

30–7. Sonohysterography is useful in which of the following conditions?

    a. endometrial polyps
    b. serosal leiomyomas
    c. septate uterus
    d. all of the above

30–8. In a 44-year-old woman with asymptomatic, 12-week-sized uterine leiomyoma, which of the following is the appropriate treatment?

    a. hysterectomy
    b. observation
    c. gonadotropin-releasing hormone (GnRH) agonists plus add-back therapy
    d. myomectomy

30–9. Which of the following is considered appropriate therapy to control bleeding in women with large leiomyomas prior to hysterectomy?

　　a. GnRH agonists
　　b. GnRH agonists plus hormone replacement therapy (HRT) add-back
　　c. Premarin, 25 mg, intravenously
　　d. none of the above

30–10. GnRH agonists have which of the following properties?

　　a. decapeptide
　　b. reduce nonmyomatous uterine volume
　　c. reduce cell size of leiomyoma
　　d. all of the above

30–11. Which of the following techniques is appropriate for myomectomy?

　　a. posterior uterine incision
　　b. GnRH agonists postoperatively
　　c. serosal injections with 200 IU Pitressin
　　d. none of the above

30–12. The highest rates of pregnancy follow which treatment for uterine synechiae?

　　a. dilation and curettage (D&C)
　　b. hysteroscopic lysis
　　c. observation
　　d. none of the above

30–13. Which of the following techniques is most accurate in the diagnosis of adenomyosis?

　　a. pelvic exam
　　b. MRI
　　c. HSG
　　d. sonohysterography

30–14. The treatment of choice for anovulatory uterine bleeding is

　　a. D&C
　　b. Depo-Provera
　　c. oral contraceptives
　　d. all of the above

30–15. The average percentage for the development of amenorrhea following laser endometrial ablation is

　　a. 25 percent
　　b. 50 percent
　　c. 90 percent
　　d. 95 percent

30–16. At which week of fetal development are uterine and vaginal development completed?

　　a. 10
　　b. 12
　　c. 14
　　d. 16

30–17. Which of the following is associated with DES exposure in utero?

　　a. uterine hypoplasia
　　b. T-shaped uterus
　　c. constriction of uterus
　　d. all of the above

30–18. Which of the following is true regarding MRI findings in a septate uterus?

　　a. not a useful test for this disorder
　　b. two high-signal intensities are seen
　　c. useful to differentiate from bicornuate uterus
　　d. none of the above

30–19. The Tompkins surgical technique is appropriate for

　　a. arcuate uterus
　　b. uterus didelphys
　　c. unicornuate uterus
　　d. none of the above

30–20. What is the dose of Pitressin (vasopressin) diluted in 20 ml of normal saline for injection in the uterus prior to reconstructive surgery?

　　a. 0.2 IU
　　b. 2.0 IU
　　c. 20 IU
　　d. 200 IU

30–21. In the Strassman procedure for a bicornuate uterus, what is the direction of the initial uterine incision?

    a. vertical
    b. transverse
    c. wedge shaped
    d. none of the above

30–22. Which of the following distending media is NOT indicated during operative hysteroscopy?

    a. Hyskon
    b. saline
    c. CO_2
    d. glycine

30–23. Which of the following syndromes is applied to uterine synechiae?

    a. Ackerman
    b. Asherman
    c. Kallmann
    d. none of the above

30–24. Diagnosis of intrauterine adhesions can be confirmed by which of the following?

    a. D&C
    b. HSG
    c. hysteroscopy
    d. all of the above

30–25. Intrauterine adhesions most commonly occur following a D&C for which of the following?

    a. menorrhagia
    b. incomplete abortion
    c. term delivery
    d. none of the above

30–26. Which of the following treatments cures adenomyosis?

    a. GnRH agonists
    b. surgical excision
    c. oral contraceptives
    d. none of the above

30–27. Abnormal bleeding in ovulatory women is often due to

    a. proliferative endometrium
    b. endometrial hyperplasia
    c. uterine leiomyoma
    d. endometrial cancer

Chapter 31
DIAGNOSIS AND MANAGEMENT OF TUBAL DISEASE

CASE REPORT

The patient is a 35-year-old white female, para 0-0-2-0, with a 3-year history of infertility. She has a history of regular periods, no history of pelvic infections or intrauterine device, and has never had reproductive surgery. Workup includes a normal semen analysis, hysterosalpingogram (HSG), and laparoscopy, yet she has an endometrial biopsy consistent with anovulation. An endocrine evaluation includes normal prolactin (PRL), thyroid-stimulating hormone (TSH), and free thyroxin levels.

She was treated with clomiphene citrate, 50 mg, on days 2 through 6 and conceived on the first treatment cycle. Quantitative β-chain human chorionic gonadotropin (hCG) on cycle day 37 was 1987 mIU/ml; on cycle day 39, the hCG titer rose to 4143 mIU/ml, and at that time an intrauterine gestational sac was visualized via transvaginal sonography. On cycle day 45, she returned for repeat scan; an intrauterine pregnancy was seen, with a crown–rump length of 0.5 cm and positive cardiac activity. However, a 3.0 × 6.1 × 4.3-cm mass was noted to the right of the midline with a 0.8-cm cystic component. No sac was identified in this structure, and a small amount of free peritoneal fluid was visualized. The patient also complained of some vague discomfort but no bleeding.

Repeat evaluation over the next 12 days showed no change in the patient's condition. There was normal development of the intrauterine pregnancy, with no change in the adnexal mass. Her hematocrit also remained stable at 36 percent. On cycle day 56, she experienced acute left lower quadrant pain; on transvaginal sonography, the intrauterine gestation measured 1.6 cm, the adnexal mass measured 4.3 × 5.9 × 6.3 cm, and there was a small amount of free peritoneal fluid noted (Fig 31–1).

A diagnostic laparoscopy was performed, which revealed adhesions between the left tube and ovary and the mesentery of the bowel with a hemorrhagic mass in the cul-de-sac. An exploratory laparotomy was performed, which confirmed the laparoscopic findings and further delineated an edematous left fallopian tube without evidence of rupture. The right ovary and right adnexa were normal. After lysis of adhesions, the adnexal mass was adherent to the cul-de-sac in the area of the left uterosacral ligament. The mass was removed by blunt dissection, and homeostasis was obtained by unipolar cautery. It was believed that this represented an incomplete tubal abortion, and a left salpingectomy was performed. Pathologic examination on the left fallopian tube showed marked edema of the serosa and an organized blood clot over its surface without evidence of tubal implantation. Immature chorionic villi with proliferating trophoblasts were identified in the specimen removed from the cul-de-sac. The patient made an unremarkable hospital recovery, was discharged home on the third postoperative day, and ultimately delivered a 2640-gm male infant at 38 weeks' gestation by cesarean section performed for cephalopelvic disproportion.

139

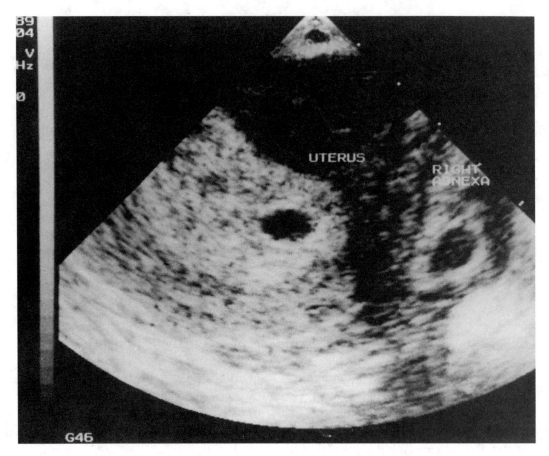

Figure 31–1. Heterotopic pregnancy diagnosed by transvaginal sonography.

SUMMARY AND CONCLUSIONS

The heterotrophic pregnancy is a rare and confounding clinical situation. This condition was virtually unheard of prior to the introduction of gonadotropin therapy with or without gamete intrafallopian transfer (GIFT) or in vitro fertilization (IVF). In fact, high-order multiple births were relatively rare prior to 1978; however, with the birth of Louise Brown, there has been an exponential rise ever since. This trend is undoubtedly due to the practice of transferring large numbers of either embryos, in the case of IVF, or oocytes, in the case of GIFT. It is suspected that with improved pregnancy rates and better insurance coverage, the practice of transferring more than 2 to 3 oocytes or embryos will become commonplace, thus lessening the possibility of heterotrophic gestations. Fortunately, modern sonography has improved our ability to diagnose these conditions, and it should al-

ways be kept in mind in the patient who presents with pain and/or bleeding and a history of superovulation.

BIBLIOGRAPHY

Gomel V, Wang I. Laparoscopic surgery for infertility therapy. *Curr Opin Obstet Gynecol.* 6:141, 1994

Lavy G, Diamond MP, DeCherney AH. Ectopic pregnancy: its relationship to tubal reconstructive surgery. *Fertil Steril.* 47:543, 1987

McComb PF, Rowe TC. Salpingitis isthmica nodosa: evidence it is a progressive disease. *Fertil Steril.* 51:542, 1989

Settlage DS, Motoshima M, Tredway DR. Sperm transport from the external cervical os to the fallopian tubes in women: a time and quantitation study. *Fertil Steril.* 24:655, 1973

Valle RF. Tubal cannulation. *Obstet Gynecol Clin North Am.* 22:519, 1995

Watson A, Vanderkerckhove P, Lilford R, et al. A meta-analysis of the therapeutic role of oil soluble contrast media at hysterosalpingography: a surprising result? *Fertil Steril.* 61:470, 1994

QUESTIONS

31–1. What is the length of the human fallopian tube?

　　a. 5 cm
　　b. 10 cm
　　c. 12 cm
　　d. 15 cm

31–2. The Müllerian ducts (paramesonephric) appear between embryonic weeks

　　a. 4 and 5
　　b. 5 and 6
　　c. 6 and 7
　　d. 7 and 8

31–3. Which of the following is true regarding the fimbria?

　　a. It is 1.5 cm in diameter.
　　b. It is 1-cm long.
　　c. There are 25 fimbriae.
　　d. all of the above

31–4. The nerve supply to the fallopian tubes comes from

　　a. T8 and T9
　　b. T10 through L2
　　c. L3 and L4
　　d. S1 and S2

31–5. Which of the following chemicals is produced by the chemical epithelium?

　　a. epidermal growth factor (EGF)
　　b. transforming growth factor-alpha (TGF-α)
　　c. leukemia inhibitory factor (LIF)
　　d. all of the above

31–6. Both fertilized and unfertilized ova remain in the ampulla for how many hours?

　　a. 24
　　b. 48
　　c. 72
　　d. 80

31–7. What portion of the ejaculated spermatozoa enter the oviduct and reach the ampulla?

　　a. 10 million
　　b. 1 million
　　c. 1000
　　d. 200

31–8. Embryos enter the uterus at which cleavage stage?

　　a. 2 cell
　　b. 4 cell
　　c. 8 to 12 cell
　　d. blastula

31–9. The incidence of congenital anomalies of the fallopian tube is

　　a. 1 in 10 million deliveries
　　b. 1 in 1 million deliveries
　　c. 1 in 500,000 deliveries
　　d. 1 in 500 deliveries

31–10. Which of the following is true regarding hydrosalpinges?

　　a. Surgery restores their patency 75 percent of the time.
　　b. The intrauterine pregnancy rate is 10 to 35 percent.
　　c. The fluid from hydrosalpinges is toxic to oocytes or embryos.
　　d. all of the above

31–11. Which of the following microorganisms have been reported to reach the fallopian tube through lymphatic and vascular channels?

　　a. *Streptococcus*
　　b. *Staphylococcus*
　　c. *Mycoplasma*
　　d. all of the above

31–12. Two episodes of pelvic inflammatory disease (PID) result in infertility how often?

　　a. 13 percent of the time
　　b. 35 percent of the time
　　c. 75 percent of the time
　　d. 100 percent of the time

31–13. Which of the following causes proximal fallopian tube obstruction?

    a. obliterative fibrosis
    b. salpingitis isthmica nodosa (SIN)
    c. uterine mural endometriosis
    d. all of the above

31–14. HSGs that demonstrate the "tobacco pouch" or "pipestem" appearance indicate tubal infection with

    a. chlamydia
    b. gonorrhea
    c. tuberculosis
    d. mycoplasma

31–15. The most successful form of tubal reanastomosis is

    a. isthmic–isthmic
    b. isthmic–ampullary
    c. ampullary–cornual
    d. ampullary–ampullary

31–16. The incidence of interstitial ectopic pregnancy is

    a. 25 percent
    b. 12 percent
    c. 5 percent
    d. 2 percent

31–17. What is the pregnancy rate following a second neosalpingostomy?

    a. 5 percent
    b. 10 percent
    c. 15 percent
    d. 20 percent

31–18. What is the rate of patency following surgery carried out on hydrosalpinges?

    a. 25 percent
    b. 50 percent
    c. 75 percent
    d. 100 percent

31–19. What is the intrauterine pregnancy rate in patients undergoing surgery for hydrosalpinges?

    a. 75 percent
    b. 50 percent
    c. 10 to 35 percent
    d. 5 percent

31–20. Which of the following is true regarding the infectious organisms that cause PID?

    a. Gonorrhea is the most common cause of the organism.
    b. Most PID is polymicrobial.
    c. *Chlamydia trachomatis* is the most common pathogen.
    d. Group A streptococcus is the most common pathogen.

31–21. Proximal tubal obstruction can be caused by

    a. tubal or cornual polyps
    b. tuberculosis
    c. remnants of chorionic ectopic pregnancy
    d. all of the above

31–22. Which of the following is true regarding intramural endometriosis?

    a. Fertility outcome after tubocornual reanastomosis is excellent.
    b. There is a low reocclusion rate following tubocornual reanastomosis.
    c. Gonadotropin-releasing hormone (GnRH) analog therapy has not been found to be effective in causing recanalization.
    d. The incidence of intramural endometriosis is 7 to 14 percent.

31–23. Which of the following is true regarding genital tuberculosis?

    a. It is usually highly symptomatic in the early stages.
    b. It presents with secondary infertility 94 percent of the time.

c. Its incidence is 20 percent in developing countries.

d. Its incidence is 10 percent among infertile women in the United States.

31–24. The disease that has been most commonly reported with falloposcopy is

a. stenosis
b. obstruction
c. intraluminal nonobstructive adhesions
d. polyps

31–25. Tubal disease accounts for what percentage of infertility?

a. 25 percent
b. 40 percent
c. 50 percent
d. 5 percent

31–26. Transcervical tubal cannulation has been reported to be successful in what percentage of patients?

a. 25 percent
b. 50 percent
c. 75 percent
d. 87 percent

31–27. During transvaginal sonography, what is the earliest date from the last menstrual period that an intrauterine gestation can be visualized?

a. 27 days
b. 35 days
c. 40 days
d. 45 days

Chapter 32

DIAGNOSIS AND MANAGEMENT OF ENDOMETRIOSIS

CASE REPORT

A 30-year-old African-American woman, G2P2, presented with a 4-month history of a painful mass in her surgical incision. She had delivered a second pregnancy by cesarean section for a complete breech presentation, followed by a tubal ligation. Her immediate postoperative course was uncomplicated. She first noted the mass 2 months later. Upon questioning, she provided information that the size of the mass and the degree of severe pain coincided with the onset of menstrual bleeding. She has no dysmenorrhea and no other symptomatic complaints. The physical findings were focused on the abdomen and the firm 2-cm mass, which was palpable within the incision (Fig 32–1). Based on the presentation, it was believed that this may represent endometriosis or suture abscess. The patient underwent a wide local incision that extended into the fascia and was primarily repaired. The follow-up revealed no recurrence at 1 year. The pathologic finding was that of endometriosis (Fig 32–2).

SUMMARY AND CONCLUSIONS

Endometriosis can be found in a number of unusual sites distal from the pelvis (Table 32–1). In fact, endometriosis has been found in males receiving high-dose estrogen therapy for prostate cancer. In the present case, it is believed that the endometrium was disrupted in large quantities during a cesarean section, which contaminated the wound.

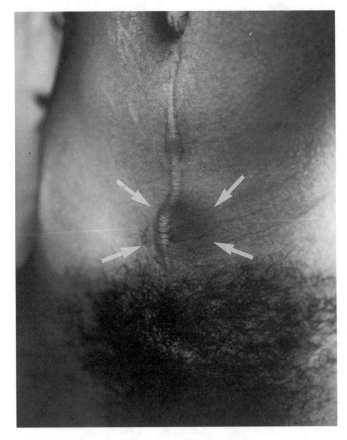

Figure 32–1. Incisional mass outlined by white arrows.

It is believed that, in genetically prone or immunologically deficient individuals, endometriosis may develop. Cases of extrauterine/pelvic endometriosis will also respond to gonadotropin-releasing hormone (GnRH) agonists. It is possible that, without prolonged medical suppression, recurrence in distal sites may follow surgery.

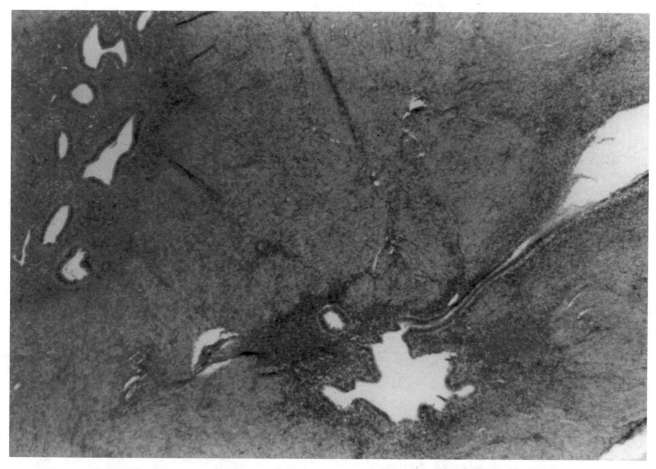

Figure 32–2. Histologic section of mass demonstrating glands and stroma, typical of endometriosis.

Table 32–1. Possible Locations of Endometriosis

Most common:	Ovary
Common:	Peritoneum of posterior cul-de-sac, uterosacral ligaments, round ligaments, oviducts and mesosalpinx, peritoneum of anterior cul-de-sac, rectosigmoid
Less common:	Cecum, appendix, bladder, vagina, small bowel, lymph nodes, omentum
Rare:	Umbilicus, laparotomy or episiotomy scars, inguinal canal, vulva, Gartner's duct, ureter, spinal canal, kidney, breast, pleura, lung, bronchus, arm, hand, thigh, spleen, heart

BIBLIOGRAPHY

Hurst BS, Schlaff WD. Treatment options for endometriosis: medical therapies. In: Diamond MP, DeCherney AH, Olive DL, eds. *Infertility and Reproductive Medicine Clinics of North America*. Philadelphia, PA, W. B. Saunders, 1992: 645–655

Jenkins S. Olive DL, Haney AF. Endometriosis: pathogenetic implications of the anatomic distribution. *Obstet Gynecol.* 67:335, 1986

Metzger DA, Haney AF. Endometriosis: etiology and pathophysiology of infertility. *Clin Obstet Gynecol.* 31:801, 1988

Schenken RS. Pathogenesis of endometriosis. In: Diamond MP, DeCherney AH, Olive DL, eds. *Infertility and Reproductive Medicine Clinics of North America*. Philadelphia, PA, W. B. Saunders, 1992: 531–544

Schrodt GR, Alcorn MD, Ibanez J. Endometriosis of the male urinary system: a case report. *J Urol.* 124:722, 1980

QUESTIONS

32–1. Endometriosis is less common in

   a. women with polycystic ovarian disease
   b. African-American women
   c. Oriental women
   d. none of the above

32–2. What percentage of women experience retrograde flow of blood into the peritoneal cavity during menses?

   a. 5 percent
   b. 25 percent
   c. 50 percent
   d. 90 percent

32–3. What percentage of women undergoing la-paroscopic tubal ligation have endometriosis?

   a. 2 percent
   b. 8 percent
   c. 15 percent
   d. 80 percent

32–4. Which of the following is true regarding pelvic pain/dysmenorrhea associated with endometriosis?

   a. There is a close correlation with the stage of disease.
   b. It is easily treated.
   c. It always disappears following meno-pause.
   d. none of the above

32–5. Which of the following is most useful in diagnosing endometriosis?

   a. CA-125
   b. magnetic resonance imaging (MRI)
   c. laparoscopy
   d. ultrasound

32–6. Which of the following are consistent with laparoscopic diagnosis of endometriosis?

   a. powder burns
   b. white plaques
   c. peritoneal pockets
   d. all of the above

32–7. Endometriomas consist of which of the fol-lowing histologic patterns?

   a. endometrial glands
   b. endometrial stroma
   c. simple cuboidal epithelium
   d. intact red blood cells

32–8. The various classification systems for en-dometriosis include all of the following EXCEPT

   a. based on clinical opinion
   b. sites of adhesions are assigned points
   c. staging based on severity of symptoms
   d. staging based on fertility prognosis

32–9. Endometriotic lesions may cause noncyclic pain by which of the following mecha-nisms?

   a. stretching of the surrounding periton-eum
   b. leaking endometriomas cause periton-eal irritation
   c. dysuria by invasion of the bladder
   d. all of the above

32–10. Which of the following is most correct?

   a. Ten percent of infertile women have endometriosis.
   b. Infertility is common in women with endometriosis.
   c. Endometriosis causes infertility.
   d. all of the above

32–11. In which of the following has their been reasonable evidence that endometriosis caused the disorder?

   a. luteal-phase defect
   b. recurrent abortion
   c. luteinized unruptured follicles (LUFs)
   d. none of the above

32–12. Danazol is characterized by which of the following?

   a. is a 19-nor-progestogen
   b. suppresses midcycle luteinizing hor-mone (LH) surge
   c. improves pregnancy rates
   d. all of the above

32–13. Which of the following is true regarding medroxyprogesterone acetate treatment in women with endometriosis?

   a. reduces dysmenorrhea
   b. associated with breakthrough bleeding
   c. fails to increase pregnancy rates
   d. all of the above

32–14. Which of the following is true regarding GnRH agonist treatment of endometriosis?

   a. reduces pain greater than danazol
   b. does not improve pregnancy rates
   c. causes a pseudopregnancy state
   d. none of the above

32–15. All of the following are true regarding in vitro fertilization and embryo transfer (IVF-ET) and endometriosis EXCEPT

    a. it requires more ampules of gonadotropin than tubal obstruction

    b. pregnancy rates are similar to tubal obstruction

    c. number of embryos are similar to tubal obstruction

    d. miscarriage rates are similar to tubal obstruction

32–16. In which of the following locations has endometriosis been reported?

    a. appendix

    b. lung

    c. spinal canal

    d. all of the above

32–17. Which of the following theories explains endometriosis in a laparotomy incision?

    a. coelomic metaplasia

    b. lymphatic dissemination

    c. retrograde menstruation

    d. none of the above

32–18. Which of the following colors is most commonly seen in older endometriosis lesions?

    a. clear

    b. red

    c. black

    d. white

32–19. Which of the following colors of endometriotic lesions are seen in younger women and are thought to represent new lesions?

    a. white

    b. clear

    c. red

    d. blue

32–20. In the American Fertility Society (AFS) classification of endometriosis, a score of 36 would be assigned to which of the following stages?

    a. I

    b. II

    c. III

    d. IV

32–21. What is the tissue source of PP14?

    a. bone marrow

    b. spleen

    c. ovary

    d. endometrial stroma

32–22. In what percentage of peritoneal pocket biopsies has endometriosis been confirmed?

    a. none

    b. 50 percent

    c. 66 percent

    d. 100 percent

32–23. The estrogen receptor content in endometriotic lesions compared to the endometrium is

    a. reduced

    b. increased compared to progesterone receptor

    c. similar

    d. none of the above

32–24. All of the following explain the etiology of pain in endometriosis EXCEPT

    a. scarring transmitted by somatic fibers of peritoneum

    b. leaking endometriosis causes peritoneal irritation

    c. uterosacral nodules transmit pain by parasympathetic innervation

    d. invasion of gut induces visceral pain

32–25. Which of the following parameters of endometriosis is NOT directly related to patient symptoms?

    a. location

    b. depth of invasion

    c. total lesion volume

    d. none of the above

32–26. Which of the following mechanisms is NOT a cause of infertility in endometriosis?

    a. cervical mucus

    b. prostaglandins

    c. autoimmunity

    d. hormonal abnormality

32–27. Which of the following treatments is indicated and shown to increase pregnancy rates in women with endometriosis?

    a. GnRH agonists

    b. mifepristone (RU 486)

    c. danazol

    d. surgery

Chapter 33

ASSISTED REPRODUCTIVE TECHNOLOGY

CASE REPORT

The patient is a 35-year-old white female, para 0-0-1-0, with a 10-year history of infertility. She underwent a myomectomy in 1992 as well as a postoperative salpingogram, which was reported as normal. Her husband was diagnosed with Crohn's disease in 1980 and was treated with 2 mg of sulfasalazine (Azulfidine) per day. He also had hypertension and was treated with 15 mg of enalapril maleate (Vasotec) per day. Prior to presenting to this assisted reproductive technology (ART) program, the patient had undergone two to three cycles of clomiphene citrate ovulation induction with intrauterine insemination (IUI) and three cycles of human menopausal gonadotropin (hMG) ovulation induction with intrauterine insemination secondary to a decreased sperm count.

She underwent an in vitro fertilization (IVF) cycle in 1992; eight eggs were retrieved and no fertilization was reported. She underwent another IVF cycle in 1993, at which time five eggs were retrieved. Partial zona dissection was used, and one egg fertilized, but no pregnancy occurred. Later that same year, she underwent IVF, and eight eggs were retrieved—four were inseminated with donor sperm and four with her husband's sperm plus partial zona dissection. Two of the husband-inseminated sperm fertilized, but none cleaved; the four donor-inseminated samples produced fertilization and cleavage but no pregnancy. Subsequently, in 1993, she underwent an additional IVF cycle with donor insemination; a biochemical pregnancy occurred. Again, in 1993, she underwent IVF with donor insemination using assisted hatching; a positive pregnancy occurred but resulted in miscarriage early in the first trimester.

In September 1993, the patient presented with a hematoperitoneum and underwent laparoscopy with subsequent laparotomy. Her hematocrit prior to surgery had decreased from 25 to 21, and her beta-human chorionic gonadotropin (β-hCG) level was reported as 18 mIU, which dropped to less than 2 mIU over the next week. The findings at the time of surgery included a large, ruptured corpus luteum cyst; multiple units of blood in the abdomen; and extensive adhesions between the left adnexa and the colon. No evidence of an ectopic pregnancy or an intrauterine pregnancy could be detected.

In December 1993, the husband's semen analysis was 17 million/mL, 41 percent motility, and 50 percent normal morphology. He also had begun to experience problems with libido and received steroid injections over 6 weeks. The patient and her husband underwent two cycles of clomiphene plus IUI, and one cycle of urofollitropin (Metrodin) plus IUI. She responded appropriately, with 1.83, 1.66, 2.0, 1.53, 1.66, and 1.33 cm follicles on day 12 and a 1.7 endometrium, and an estradiol level of 712 pg/ml. All therapeutic levels carried out since December 1993 were done with the husband off of Azulfidine, a known spermatotoxic agent.

Subsequently, the patient underwent a gamete intrafallopian transfer (GIFT) cycle using leuprolide acetate (Lupron), Metrodin 150 IV, and Pergonal 150 IV. On cycle day 11, eight mature follicles were

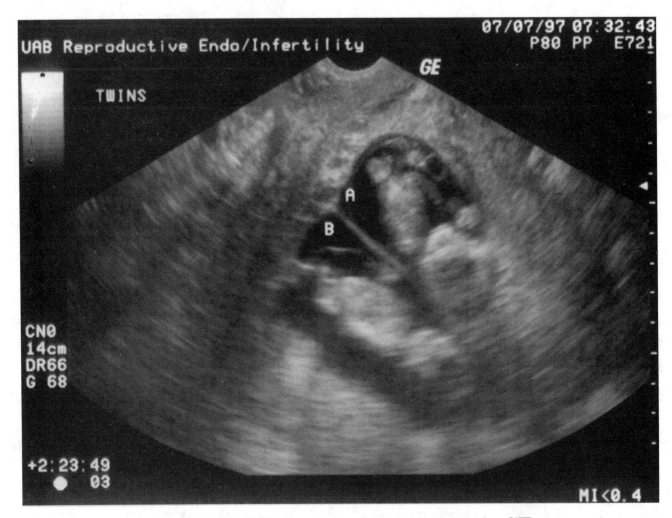

Figure 33–1. Transvaginal sonogram showing twin gestation resulting from GIFT.

present—1.93, 1.5, 1.73, 1.56, 1.53, 1.86, 1.63, and 1.83 cm—with a 1.7 cm endometrium and an estradiol level of 1053 pg/ml. GIFT was carried out in October 1994, which resulted in a viable twin gestation which ultimately went to a term delivery (Fig 33–1).

SUMMARY AND CONCLUSIONS

The failure to conceive following IVF is frustrating for both the patient and the physician. While IVF lies at one end of the therapeutic spectrum and often is treated by the patient and physician as a mechanistic process, ruled by protocol and mysticism, it should be remembered that this is but another form of medical therapy. This means that every attempt should be made to evaluate a couple thoroughly prior to proceeding with this financially and emotionally costly procedure. One of the pil-

lars of good health care dictates that couples' problems be explored with an adequate history. Numerous drugs have been found that affect male fertility, ranging from such diverse agents as cimetidine hydrochloride (Tagamet), which induces hyperprolactinemia and oligospermia, and nifedipine (Procardia), which may alter sperm–egg binding, to Azulfidine, which in this case was a deterrent to fertilization.

BIBLIOGRAPHY

Lenz S, Lauritsen JG, Kjellow M. Collection of human oocytes for IVF by ultrasonically guided follicular puncture. *Lancet*. 1:1163, 1981

Meldrum DR, Wisot A, Hamilton F, et al. Routine pituitary suppression with leuprolide before ovarian stimulation for oocyte retrieval. *Fertil Steril*. 5:455, 1989

Palermo G, Joris H, Devroey P, van Steirteghem AC. Pregnancies after intracytoplasmic injection of single spermatozoon into an oocyte. *Lancet.* 340:17, 1992

Sauer MV, Paulson RJ, Lobo RA. A preliminary report on oocyte donation extending reproductive potential to women over 40. *N Engl J Med.* 323:1157, 1990

Steptoe PC, Edwards RG. Birth after reimplantation of a human embryo. *Lancet.* 2:366, 1978

Trounsen AO, Mohn L. Human pregnancy following cryopreservation, thawing and transfer of an eight-cell embryo. *Nature.* 305:707, 1983

QUESTIONS

33–1. Tubal disease accounts for what percentage of infertility?

    a. 10 percent
    b. 25 percent
    c. 35 percent
    d. 40 percent

33–2. ART accounts for how many deliveries in the United States per year?

    a. 2000
    b. 5000
    c. 9500
    d. 15,000

33–3. What percentage of couples will achieve pregnancy within four IVF treatment cycles?

    a. 25 percent
    b. 50 percent
    c. 75 percent
    d. 100 percent

33–4. Which of the following decreases pregnancy rates following IVF?

    a. advanced maternal age
    b. the presence of hydrosalpinges
    c. male factor infertility
    d. all of the above

33–5. Which of the following is NOT a normal parameter of a semen analysis according to the World Health Organization?

    a. concentration of sperm >20 million sperm/ml
    b. motility >40 percent
    c. normal morphology >50 percent
    d. none of the above

33–6. Prior to the development of intracytoplasmic sperm injection, which sperm concentration predicted poor outcome in conventional IVF?

    a. counts <5 million
    b. counts <3 million
    c. counts <1.5 million
    d. none of the above

33–7. Which of the following is NOT true regarding diethylstilbestrol (DES) patients?

    a. They have a higher incidence of prematurity.
    b. They have the same incidence of infertility as the general population.
    c. IVF outcomes of DES patients generally are less favorable than individuals with tubal factors.
    d. They have a higher incidence of ectopic pregnancy.

33–8. The likelihood of a woman age 40 or over conceiving through IVF is

    a. 40 percent per cycle
    b. 25 percent per cycle
    c. 9 percent per cycle
    d. none of the above

33–9. Which of the following does NOT contribute to decreased fertility in women over age 40 undergoing IVF?

    a. oocyte immaturity
    b. poor ovulatory response
    c. aging of the uterine milieu
    d. none of the above

33–10. Which of the following has been used to evaluate ovarian reserve?

    a. day 3 follicle-stimulating hormone (FSH)
    b. day 3 estradiol
    c. response of FSH to clomiphene challenge
    d. all of the above

33–11. Which of the following results in an increased pregnancy rate in IVF?

    a. downregulation with gonadotropin-releasing hormone (GnRH) analogs
    b. the development of intracytoplasmic sperm injection (ICSI) technology
    c. improved methods of cryopreservation
    d. all of the above

33–12. Which of the following is used to grade oocytes?

    a. oocyte corona cumulus complex
    b. mucification and dispersal of the corona radiata
    c. presence or absence of nuclear membrane (germinal vesicle) or polar body
    d. all of the above

33–13. The mature preovulatory follicle displays which of the following?

    a. condensed cumulus and zona radiata
    b. zona pellucida not readily visualized
    c. opaque ooplasm
    d. first polar body indicating that the oocyte is in metaphase

33–14. Which of the following contributes to a successful IVF laboratory?

    a. evaluation of embryo toxicity using 2- to 4-cell mouse embryo assays
    b. using highly purified water
    c. using advanced air-handling equipment
    d. all of the above

33–15. The first birth in animals by IVF was reported in

    a. 1878
    b. 1944
    c. 1959
    d. 1978

33–16. The decline in pregnancy rate seen in older women is due to

    a. aging of the uterine milieu
    b. defective gonadotropin production
    c. an increased rate of numeric chromosomal anomalies in egg cells
    d. total depletion of oocytes

33–17. The clomiphene challenge test assesses ovarian responsiveness by

    a. generating an exaggerated rise in FSH levels
    b. generating an exaggerated rise in luteinizing hormone (LH) levels
    c. doubling the baseline estradiol levels
    d. doubling the baseline inhibin levels

33–18. The purpose of beginning GnRH analog therapy in the middle of the luteal phase is to

    a. produce a flare effect and amplify egg growth
    b. directly inhibit progesterone production
    c. selectively inhibit endogenous LH production
    d. downregulate gonadotrope GnRH receptors

33–19. The availability of clinically useful GnRH antagonists has been hampered by

    a. the cost
    b. the histaminic side effects
    c. the hydrophobic nature of molecules
    d. all of the above

33–20. The most common dose of leuprolide acetate used to inhibit LH surges is

    a. 0.25 mg
    b. 0.5 mg
    c. 1 mg
    d. 2 mg

33–21. GnRH analog flare usually lasts

    a. 2 days
    b. 5 days
    c. 7 days
    d. 10 days

33–22. Oocytes are generally retrieved how many hours following hCG administration?

    a. 24
    b. 30
    c. 34 to 36
    d. 40

33–23. What is the typical frequency of the ultrasound transducer used for transvaginal retrievals?

    a. 4 MHz
    b. 5 to 7 MHz
    c. 10 MHz
    d. 15 MHz

33–24. How many motile sperm are ordinarily added to each oocyte for insemination?

    a. 50,000
    b. 100,000 to 200,000
    c. 500,000
    d. 1 million

33–25. Which of the following is true regarding the medium used for embryo culture?

    a. The medium contains bicarbonate.
    b. It requires an atmosphere of 5 percent CO_2 for equilibration.
    c. The physiologic pH is 7.4.
    d. all of the above

33–26. The single factor that has had the greatest effect on the increasing multiple birth rates following IVF is the

    a. age of the woman
    b. improvement in culture conditions
    c. number of embryos transferred
    d. use of pure FSH ovulation induction protocols

33–27. What is the likelihood of a woman over age 40 aborting after an IVF cycle?

    a. 15 percent
    b. 20 percent
    c. 25 percent
    d. 50 percent

Chapter 34
RECURRENT PREGNANCY LOSS

CASE REPORT

A 25-year-old female, para 0-0-4-0, presented for evaluation of recurrent pregnancy loss. From age 20 to age 25, she experienced pregnancy losses of 7, 8, 12, and 12 weeks (Table 34–1). During the fourth pregnancy, she had a sonogram that revealed the possibility of a septate or bicornuate uterus. Her present husband fathered all her pregnancies. The history and physical examination was normal. Her evaluation included the following:

Hormonal:	Day 21 progesterone 18 ng/ml
	Thyroid-stimulating hormone (TSH) 7 µu/ml
Chromosomal:	Wife, 46,XX
	Husband, 46,XY
Mycoplasma and chlamydial cultures:	Negative
Lupus anticoagulant and antiphospholipid antibodies:	Negative
Hysterosalpingogram (HSG):	Septate vs bicornuate uterus (Fig 34–1)
Intravenous pyelogram (IVP):	Normal

Table 34–1. Pregnancy History

Age	Weeks	Preg Test	Sono-sac	FHT	Outcome
20	7	+	ND	ND	D&C
21	8	+	ND	ND	Complete AB
22	12	+	+	+	Complete AB
25	12	+	Sac/?bicornuate	+	D&C

ND = not detected and/or sono not obtained; FHT = fetal heart tone; AB = abortion; D&C = dilation and curettage.

After a discussion with the patient, a decision to proceed with laparoscopy and/or hysteroscopy was made.

At the time of the laparoscopy, a bicornuate uterus was seen. A laparotomy incision was performed, and a Strassman metroplasty was performed to unify the two uterine horns (see Fig 30–12 of *Textbook of Reproductive Medicine*, 2nd ed., for techniques used). At 3 months following surgery, a repeat HSG was performed, which demonstrated significant improvement with a larger single cavity (Fig 34–2).

At 5 months following surgery, the patient conceived and delivered a liveborn infant at 38 weeks by primary cesarean section.

SUMMARY AND CONCLUSIONS

A bicornuate uterus is much less common than a septate uterus. The treatment of a septate uterus is relatively simple and involves day surgery and hysteroscopic resection. In contrast, bicornuate surgery requires a laparotomy, risk of uterine rupture during a subsequent pregnancy, and an elective cesarean section for delivery. The rate of pregnancy loss prior to surgery for bicornuate uterus ranges from 15 to 75 percent. For this reason, prior to a surgical repair for a bicornuate uterus, demonstration of at least three pregnancy losses is strongly suggested. Surgical repair reduces pregnancy loss by 20 to 50 percent.

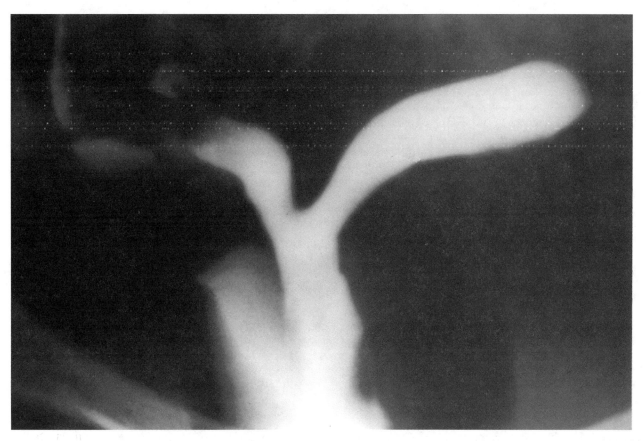

Figure 34–1. Preoperative HSG revealing possible bicornuate versus septate uterus.

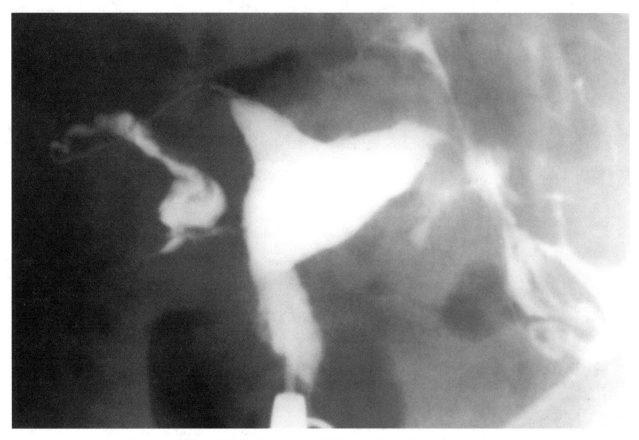

Figure 34–2. Postoperative HSG revealing unified cavity.

BIBLIOGRAPHY

American Fertility Society. The American Fertility Society classifications of adnexal adhesions, distal tubal occlusion, tubal occlusion secondary to tubal ligation, tubal pregnancies, Müllerian anomalies and intrauterine adhesions. *Fertil Steril.* 49:944, 1988

Buttram VC, Gibbons WE. Müllerian anomalies: a proposed classification (an analysis of 144 cases). *Fertil Steril.* 32:40, 1979

Cooper JM, Houck RM, Rigberg HS. The incidence of intrauterine abnormalities found at hysteroscopy in patients undergoing elective hysteroscopic sterilization. *J Reprod Med.* 28:659, 1983

Greiss FC, Mauzy CH. Genital anomalies in women: an evaluation of diagnosis, incidence and obstetrical performance. *Am J Obstet Gynecol.* 82:330, 1961

Portuondo JA, Clmara MM, Echanojauregui AD, et al. Müllerian abnormalities in fertile women and recurrent aborters. *J Reprod Med.* 31:616, 1986

Rock JA. Diagnosing and repairing uterine anomalies. *Contemp Obstet Gynecol.* 1:17, 1981

Rock JA, Jones HW Jr. The clinical management of the double uterus. *Fertil Steril.* 28:798, 1977

QUESTIONS

34–1. Which of the following describes a preclinical loss of a pregnancy?

   a. failure of egg division
   b. failure of implantation
   c. blastocyst lost with subsequent menstruation
   d. all of the above

34–2. Of the 25 percent of women who experience spotting in early pregnancy, what percentage of these women deliver at term?

   a. 25 percent
   b. 50 percent
   c. 75 percent
   d. 90 percent

34–3. If an embryo demonstrates a crown–rump length of 5 to 9 mm and a fetal heart rate (FHR) of 90, which of the following is correct?

   a. Repeat ultrasound at 20 weeks.
   b. A poor outcome is predicted.
   c. FHR at this stage is not predictive of outcome.
   d. none of the above

34–4. If both the preclinical and clinical pregnancy loss are considered, what is the overall total rate of loss?

   a. 10 to 15 percent
   b. 15 to 25 percent
   c. 20 to 30 percent
   d. 30 to 40 percent

34–5. If a couple has never delivered a liveborn infant but has experienced four repeat early pregnancy losses of unknown etiology, what is their chance of having a liveborn child?

   a. 25 percent
   b. 50 percent
   c. 75 percent
   d. 80 percent

34–6. What is the most common cause of repeat pregnancy loss?

   a. endocrine
   b. infection
   c. genetic
   d. anatomic

34–7. What is the most common chromosomal anomaly in first trimester spontaneous abortions?

   a. trisomy
   b. triploidy
   c. translocations
   d. none of the above

34–8. What percentage of women with repeat pregnancy loss are found to have intrauterine synechiae?

   a. 5 percent
   b. 10 percent
   c. 15 percent
   d. 45 percent

34–9. What is the incidence of lupus anticoagulant or anticardiolipin (aCL) antibody in a low-risk population without previous pregnancy loss?

   a. 2 percent
   b. 4 percent
   c. 8 percent
   d. 20 percent

34–10. Which of the following tests is used to screen for lupus anticoagulant?

   a. aCL antibody
   b. immunoglobulin G (IgG)
   c. kaolin clotting time (KCT)
   d. antinuclear antibody (ANA)

34–11. Which of the following treatments has been shown clearly to be effective in reducing pregnancy loss in women with high levels of lupus anticoagulant and high levels of aCL antibody?

   a. intravenous immunoglobulin
   b. prednisone
   c. aspirin plus heparin
   d. all of the above

34–12. Leukocyte immunization

   a. has not been clinically proven useful for alloimmune causes of repeat pregnancy loss
   b. is a paternal source of leukocytes
   c. is a maternal source of leukocytes
   d. all of the above

34–13. Infectious agents associated with repeat early pregnancy loss include

   a. *Mycoplasma hominis*
   b. group A streptococcus
   c. tuberculosis
   d. *Staphylococcus aureus*

34–14. Evaluation of an endocrine cause of repeat pregnancy loss includes all of the following EXCEPT

   a. follicle-stimulating hormone (FSH)
   b. TSH
   c. prolactin
   d. midluteal progesterone

34–15. A 22-year-old patient with two consecutive pregnancy losses and no live births presents for evaluation and treatment. What do you tell or order for this patient?

   a. 50 percent chance of next pregnancy being a live birth
   b. refer to a specialist for genetic counseling

   c. day 18 endometrial biopsy
   d. none of the above

34–16. In what percentage of couples after a basic evaluation for recurrent pregnancy loss can an etiology be determined?

   a. 30 percent
   b. 60 percent
   c. 80 percent
   d. 95 percent

34–17. What is the incidence of chromosomal anomalies in liveborn infants?

   a. 5 percent
   b. 2.5 percent
   c. 1.5 percent
   d. 0.5 percent

34–18. In what percentage of couples can a balanced translocation or other chromosomal abnormality be detected as a cause of recurrent pregnancy loss?

   a. 1 percent
   b. 3 percent
   c. 10 percent
   d. 12 percent

34–19. Which of the following methods are utilized to treat luteal-phase defects?

   a. bromocriptine
   b. human chorionic gonadotropin
   c. clomiphene
   d. all of the above

34–20. What is the incidence of Müllerian anomalies in women with normal reproductive histories?

   a. 1 percent
   b. 5 percent
   c. 10 percent
   d. 15 percent

34–21. Diethylstilbestrol (DES) exposure is associated with all of the following EXCEPT

   a. term pregnancy
   b. ectopic pregnancy
   c. improved pregnancy rates after metroplasty
   d. spontaneous abortion

34–22. Which of the following is the preferred surgical method for a bicornuate uterus?

    a. operative hysteroscopy by laser
    b. operative hysteroscopy by scissors
    c. Strassman
    d. Tompkins

34–23. Alloimmune theories proposed to explain fetal loss include

    a. CD 56-negative natural killer cells
    b. T-suppressor cells
    c. antipaternal cytotoxic antibodies
    d. all of the above

34–24. Which of the following tests are used to screen for lupus anticoagulant?

    a. dilute Russell viper venom time (dRVVT)
    b. prothrombin time
    c. concentrated viper venom time
    d. all of the above

34–25. Human leukocyte antigen (HLA) typing of couples with repeat pregnancy loss is associated with which of the following?

    a. requires donor sperm
    b. abnormal test includes increased sharing of loci

    c. treated successfully with immunoglobulin
    d. all of the above

34–26. What percentage of referral populations of women with recurrent loss have detectable antiphospholipid antibodies?

    a. 1 percent
    b. 3 percent
    c. 7 percent
    d. 15 percent

34–27. The antiphospholipid syndrome (APS) requires which of the following laboratory tests to be positive on at least two occasions?

    a. lupus anticoagulant
    b. IgG anticardiolipin antibodies
    c. IgM anticardiolipin antibodies
    d. all of the above

INFERTILITY AND PREGNANCY LOSS: PSYCHOLOGICAL ASPECTS OF TREATMENT

Chapter 35

CASE REPORT

The patient is a 29-year-old white female, para 0-0-0-0, who presented in November 1985. Her previous workup had consisted of a negative hysterosalpingogram (HSG), a normal semen analysis, and laparoscopy which showed stage III endometriosis by the original American Fertility Society criteria. Subsequently, she was treated preoperatively with 6 months of danazol and then underwent exploratory laparotomy and resection of endometriosis, lysis of adhesions, resection of an endometrioma, and appendectomy. She was treated with Hyskon (dextran-70 in dextrose) intraoperatively as an antiadhesive agent. She has received no further therapy since March 1986.

Significant past medical history included that her husband had fathered one child by a previous marriage. The physical examination showed a well-nourished female with a weight of 126 lb, height 5'6", blood pressure 108/64, pulse 66, and respirations 12. No thyromegaly was noted, nor was galactorrhea. Pelvic examination was normal. She received a diagnosis of endometriosis and was treated with Tylenol #3 (acetaminophen and codeine) and Anaprox (naproxen sodium) for menstrual cramps. She was scheduled for a midluteal progesterone level, timed sonography, postcoital test, and culture for mycoplasma. A postcoital test done on cycle day

12, timed to a basal body temperature chart, showed clear abundant mucus with 6-cm spinnbarkeit and 6 to 8 directionally motile sperm/ hpf. Her serum progesterone level was 8 ng/ml, and follicle scanning done prior to ovulation showed multiple small follicles of approximately 1.2 cm in size on cycle day 12. Her prolactin and thyroid-stimulating hormone (TSH) levels were normal, and she was started on clomiphene citrate, 50 mg, on days 2 through 6.

At about this juncture, she began to have increasing menstrual cramps, was changed to ibuprofen (Motrin), and in March 1986 began to experience pain at the time of ovulation and pain with intercourse. She was treated with a total of four cycles of clomiphene citrate, with progesterone levels being recorded greater than 15 ng/ml and adequate follicle development. Subsequently, she underwent a second look laparoscopy in June 1986. Hysteroscopic examination revealed a normal uterine cavity and patent bilateral tubal ostia. The right ovary was found to be attached to the pelvic sidewall with filmy adhesions, and these were lysed without difficulty. The left tube and ovary were normal. There was scarring in the cul-de-sac consistent with old endometriosis. The uterus was fixed anteriorly secondary to a previous uterine suspension. The left fallopian tube was seen lateral to the ovary, which was cystic in nature, and adhesions were present, binding it to the colon. Clear fluid was aspirated from the cyst, indicating that it was not an endometrioma. The fallopian tubes were patent bilaterally to chromotubation with indigo carmine.

Following the second look procedure, the patient was continued on ovulation induction with clomiphene, ultimately at a dose of 150 mg/day. In August 1986, the patient was treated with Pergonal superovulation induction; she had an adequate response on 150 mIU/day and ovulated successfully in two consecutive cycles. In November 1986, she began to have further marital problems associated with infertility, at which time she went into counseling and discontinued therapy for one month. In December 1986, she was restarted on Pergonal therapy and was treated with two further cycles. In August 1987, the patient presented complaining with pain on the left side for a week's duration. Sonogram revealed a $2.8 \times 2.8 \times 2.6$-cm cystic structure. She was 4 days late for menstruation. Pelvic examination revealed a fixed, irregular uterus. A pregnancy test was negative. She was begun on norethindrone acetate therapy for recurrent pelvic pain, presumably secondary to endometriosis. Norethindrone acetate therapy relieved her pelvic pain, and she was not troubled with hot flashes but was lethargic and experienced breakthrough bleeding, and the therapy was discontinued in February 1989. She had taken a total of 6 months' treatment course. By September 1989, she was having recurrent symptoms compatible with endometriosis: dyspareunia, sacral pain at the time of menstruation, and interior thigh pain. Discussion was carried out regarding leuprolide acetate (Lupron) therapy, norethindrone acetate therapy, or treatment with birth control pills. She elected not to take any suppressive medication and wished to try for pregnancy without therapy. In September 1990, she returned with increasing menstrual cramps, was treated with meclofenamate sodium (Meclomen), and counseling was carried out regarding in vitro fertilization. In November 1991, she was beginning to have severe menstrual cramps and dyspareunia. She again declined therapy with either Lupron or norethindrone acetate, and by September 1992, she had become separated from her husband, her body weight had dropped to 121 lb, and she developed irregular menstruation and increased cramps. She was treated with Loestrin (norethindrone acetate and ethinyl estradiol) 1/20 for control of menstrua-

tion and ketorolac (Toradol) for pain. Following her divorce, she moved to a neighboring state in May 1993 to enter into a business arrangement with her sister. She had developed a new relationship and her mental status had markedly improved. By January 1996, she had remarried and discontinued all hormonal therapy; when last seen in June 1997, she had returned to her original body weight, had reconciled her lack of childbearing, and was prepared to enter into discussion regarding the perimenopausal life transition.

SUMMARY AND CONCLUSIONS

Patients who are undergoing infertility therapy or have experienced pregnancy loss are under tremendous social and self-imposed pressures. Society and the family demand that couples reproduce to "preserve the family name," but in reality, this represents no more than the drive of genes to replicate. Couples who fail to conceive begin to question life, its meaning, and their role in it. At times, the drive to conceive becomes an obsession, at least with one member of the couple. As a result of this, all aspects of the marriage become captive to the process of reproduction. Although infertile couples do remarkably well in terms of most aspects of their lives, they are unfortunately more susceptible to divorce than the population at large. If one in two couples divorce in the population as a whole, the situation with the infertile couple is worse. This may be a natural response, as one would assume if conception cannot occur with one partner, it may well occur with another. When one considers that the state of subfertility is a balance between male and female reproductive potential, this may in fact be true. However, the clinician must be careful to expedite the evaluation and treatment program and always be vigilant for unstated marital difficulties that may respond to appropriate counseling.

BIBLIOGRAPHY

McCormick RM. Out of control: one apsect of infertility. *J Obstet Gynecol Neonat Nurs.* 1:105, 1980

Peppers L, Knapp R. Maternal reaction to involuntary fetal/infant death. *Psychiatry.* 43:155, 1980

Rosenfeld DL, Mitchell E. Treating the emotional aspects of infertility: counseling services in an infertility clinic. *Am J Obstet Gynecol.* 135:177, 1979

Seibel MM, Taymor ML. Emotional aspects of infertility. *Fertil Steril.* 37:137, 1982

QUESTIONS

35–1. Patients may respond to infertility or pregnancy loss with

   a. denial
   b. anger
   c. withdrawal
   d. all of the above

35–2. Which of the following therapies has proven useful for the treatment of infertility?

   a. adoption
   b. relaxation
   c. discontinuation of therapy
   d. none of the above

35–3. The inability to conceive challenges

   a. self-value
   b. self-concept
   c. marital stability
   d. all of the above

35–4. Which of the following reactions is common when bodily malfunctions are detected during the infertility workup?

   a. blame
   b. guilt
   c. fear of rejection
   d. all of the above

35–5. The most stress-provoking factor in infertility is

   a. loss of time
   b. the expense of therapy
   c. loss of control over one's body
   d. family rejection

35–6. Production of a semen analysis by masturbation arouses feelings of

   a. guilt
   b. inadequacy
   c. anxiety
   d. all of the above

35–7. Which of the following is true regarding the behavior of infertile couples?

   a. They are comfortable around other couples' children.
   b. They are comfortable attending social functions such as baby showers.
   c. They mix easily with obstetric patients at the physician's office.
   d. none of the above

35–8. A significant problem that can occur in association with a postcoital test is

   a. inconvenient timing of intercourse
   b. premature ejaculation
   c. impotence
   d. poor outcome

35–9. When compared with the population at large, infertile couples have

   a. more financial problems
   b. a greater incidence of sexual dysfunction
   c. a higher incidence of divorce
   d. none of the above

35–10. The initial workup indicates that infertility is treatable in couples who do not experience

   a. hope
   b. apprehension and frustration
   c. conflict
   d. none of the above

35–11. The least satisfactory way of concluding infertility treatment is

   a. pregnancy
   b. dropout
   c. to re-evaluate and restructure the couple's life
   d. to enter perimenopause

35–12. Adoption does not satisfy the need to

   a. become parents
   b. be pregnant
   c. conclude the infertility therapy
   d. resolve stress between the couple

35–13. Which of the following characterizes the grief process?

    a. denial
    b. isolation and anger
    c. grief and resolution
    d. all of the above

35–14. It is estimated that stress causes what percentage of infertility?

    a. 2 percent
    b. 10 percent

    c. 50 percent
    d. 90 percent

35–15. Language that aggravates the fault/blame tendency in infertile couples includes

    a. incompetent cervix
    b. failed cycle
    c. ovarian failure
    d. all of the above

VI

CONTRACEPTION

Chapter 36

CONTRACEPTION

CASE REPORT

The patient is a 20-year-old white female, para 0–0–2–0, with abortions in 1993 and 1995. She presents with severe dysmenorrhea and abnormal uterine bleeding since receiving an injection of medroxyprogesterone acetate (Depo-Provera 150) for contraception and the control of pelvic pain. She has a history of mitral valve prolapse with dysautonomia and takes fludrocortisone acetate (Florinef) and amitriptyline, as well as phenobarbital and clonazepam (Klonopin) for a seizure disorder. It should be noted that her dysautonomic syndrome markedly worsened since receiving Depo-Provera. Prior to receiving this, she had been weaned off her dysautonomic medications and was under good control. Since that time, she has developed symptoms of weakness, orthostatic changes, periodic tachycardia, pallor, sleep disturbance, and lethargy. She had a history of 30-day, regular menstrual cycles, with bleeding lasting 4 to 5 days and requiring 4 to 5 pads per day.

Her past medical history is further significant in that she underwent a laparoscopy in 1994 for an ovarian cyst and had a paraganglioma removed in 1991. She requires medication such as Percodan (oxycodone hydrochloride, oxycodone terephthalate, and aspirin) for control of her dysmenorrhea, and she has a history of herpes simplex and genital warts. She is a student and has a history of alcohol, tobacco, and recreational drug use. As noted previously, she has had two abortions for unplanned pregnancies.

Physical examination shows a thin white female, 5′4″ in height, 114 lb, with a blood pressure of 120/74. She presents lying in the fetal position on the examining table. The remainder of her physical examination is unremarkable with the exception of a midsystolic click noted on inspiration.

She was begun on a protocol of 1-mg estradiol (Estrace) on days 1 through 25 and 5 mg of norethindrone acetate on days 16 through 25. She was seen for followup a month later and had some breakthrough bleeding. It should be noted that her dysautonomia was under control, and the norethindrone acetate was increased to 10 mg/day.

SUMMARY AND CONCLUSIONS

This particular patient presents with several features that are compatible with chronic pain syndrome and complications associated with injectable contraceptive agents. First, she has two medical problems; that is, seizures and mitral valve prolapse with dysautonomia, which are at times disabling for her. She has severe dysmenorrhea that does not have a clear etiology, and, unfortunately, the administration of Depo-Provera worsened the overall situation. We have seen many patients with dysautonomic syndrome who have an exacerbation of their symptoms during the luteal phase when exposed to progestogens. Further, in patients who are amenorrheic with this disorder, stability is easily obtained with estrogen alone; however, progestogens invariably cause some exacerbation. Further, Depo-Provera, when administered to any woman, can produce ovulatory dysfunction for up to 2 years. A single dose of Depo-Provera at 25 mg can induce ovulatory dysfunction for at least 12 months. The fact that this patient is at minimal body weight at 114 lb, with a height of 5′4″, and has an inappropriate fat–lean mass ratio, predisposes her to ovulatory dysfunction.

An attempt was made to treat this patient with low-dose birth control pills in the past; however, it should be remembered that the birth control pill containing ethinyl estradiol in the range of 20 µg to 35 µg does not suppress folliculogenesis but only

165

blocks ovulation, and the biological action is dependent upon a certain production of endogenous estrone and 17β-estradiol. It is quite common for patients with altered lean mass–body fat ratios to respond poorly to low-dose birth control pills and become amenorrheic or develop abnormal uterine bleeding. In a patient with an already suppressed uterine lining, the addition of a drug such as Depo-Provera will often produce protracted uterine lining instability and bleeding. This patient's response to her overall condition as well as her past medical history suggests immaturity, a certain antisocial personality, and inadequate self-discipline. Her ultimate solution to this problem was to seek hysterectomy from another gynecologist at age 20.

BIBLIOGRAPHY

Devereux RB, Kramer-Fox L, Klingfield P. Mitral valve prolapse causes clinical manifestations in management. *Ann Int Med.* 111:305, 1989

Frisch RE, McArthur JS. Menstrual cycles: fatness as a determinant of minimum weight or height necessary for their maintenance or onset. *Science.* 185:949, 1974

Levy D, Savage DD. Prevalence in clinical features of mitral valve prolapse: The Framingham Study. *Am Heart J.* 113:1281, 1987

QUESTIONS

36–1. Typical first-year accidental pregnancy rate for condom use is

   a. 7 percent
   b. 12 percent
   c. 17 percent
   d. 19 percent

36–2. The contraceptive sponge is

   a. made of latex and polyethylene
   b. associated with first-year accidental pregnancy rates of 11 percent
   c. effective for 48 hours
   d. not associated with toxic shock syndrome

36–3. All of the following are true regarding the intrauterine device (IUD) EXCEPT

   a. they are used by 85 million worldwide
   b. they are used by 25 million worldwide

   c. they are associated with low pregnancy rates
   d. copper IUDs are associated with increased menstrual blood loss

36–4. Which of the following is true regarding IUDs?

   a. Progestasert contains 38 mg of levonorgestrel.
   b. The copper IUD currently marketed in the United States has no copper on the horizontal arms.
   c. The copper IUD is associated with low rates of ectopic pregnancy.
   d. none of the above

36–5. Which of the following is recommended if pregnancy occurs in a woman with an IUD?

   a. remove if string visible
   b. patient informed of increased risk of pregnancy-related complications
   c. consider abortion if string not visible
   d. all of the above

36–6. What percentage of men having a vasectomy develop antibodies to sperm?

   a. 0 percent
   b. 10 percent
   c. 50 percent
   d. 100 percent

36–7. Which of the following is true regarding the rhythm method of contraception?

   a. used by 20 percent of couples
   b. associated with a first-year accidental pregnancy rate of 10 percent
   c. needs to be used only during days 12 through 16 of cycle
   d. efficacy is improved with luteinizing hormone (LH) predictor kits

36–8. Which of the following is true regarding the oral contraceptive pill?

a. The progestin component regulates bleeding.
b. The estrogen component inhibits ovulation.
c. The primary mechanism of action is inhibition of gonadotropins.
d. all of the above

36–9. Which of the following progestogens in oral contraceptives is the most potent?

a. norethindrone
b. levonorgestrel
c. norgestimate
d. all equally potent

36–10. Which of the following is known regarding oral contraceptives and ovarian cysts?

a. less risk with triphasic
b. less risk with monophasic
c. used successfully to cause rapid regression of cysts
d. none of the above

36–11. Which of the following is a potential risk of low-dose oral contraceptives (≤35 μg ethinyl estradiol) in a 25-year-old nonsmoker?

a. thromboembolism
b. myocardial infarction
c. development of diabetes
d. none of the above

36–12. Which of the following neoplasms are reduced by oral contraceptive use?

a. colon cancer
b. ovarian cancer
c. breast cancer
d. cervical cancer

36–13. Postcoital contraception includes which of the following?

a. needs to be used within 72 hours of exposure
b. mifepristone (RU 486)

c. high-dose (50 μg ethinyl estradiol) pills
d. all of the above

36–14. The use of Depo-Provera and effects include which of the following?

a. Depo-Provera, 250 mg, IM every 3 months
b. inhibition of ovulation
c. increases high-density lipoprotein (HDL)
d. none of the above

36–15. All of the following are true regarding levonorgestrel implants EXCEPT they

a. are effective for 8 years
b. need to be removed
c. are less effective in obese women
d. can be inserted on a gluteal surface

36–16. Contraceptive techniques have been utilized for how many years according to written records?

a. 60
b. 100
c. 1000
d. 3000

36–17. In the United States, which form of reversible contraception is the most commonly utilized?

a. condom
b. sponge
c. oral contraceptives
d. none of the above

36–18. The Lea shield is

a. an IUD
b. a vaginal sponge
c. made of silicone
d. none of the above

36–19. All of the following are true regarding contraceptive creams EXCEPT that they

a. require a prescription
b. are effective when used alone
c. are spermicidal
d. prevent sexually transmitted disease

36–20. The Progestasert IUD is clinically approved for how many years?

a. 1
b. 3
c. 7
d. 10

36–21. Which of the following contraceptives contains ethynodiol diacetate?

a. Ovcon
b. Loestrin
c. Demulin
d. Desogen

36–22. Which of the following contraceptives contains norgestimate?

a. Ortho-Cept
b. Ovrette
c. both of the above
d. none of the above

36–23. Which of the following oral contraceptives is best used in lactating women?

a. Ovrette
b. Micronor
c. Nor-Q.D.
d. all of the above

36–24. If a woman who is on the pill presents with amenorrhea, which of the following is correct?

a. She is most likely pregnant.
b. She should immediately discontinue the pill.

c. A pill with a higher estrogen content can be prescribed.
d. A pill with a higher progestin content can be prescribed.

36–25. Which of the following terms describes facial pigmentation that can occur in oral contraceptive users?

a. Nelson syndrome
b. chloasma
c. Peutz–Jeghers syndrome
d. all of the above

36–26. Which of the following laboratory test values is increased in oral contraceptive users?

a. vitamin B_6
b. antithrombin III
c. vitamin A
d. all of the above

36–27. All of the following are absolute contraindications of oral contraceptive use EXCEPT

a. hypertension
b. thromboembolism
c. impaired liver function
d. history of cholestasis during pregnancy

VII

MENOPAUSE

Chapter 37

PHYSIOLOGY OF THE CLIMACTERIC

37–1. The age of menopause is delayed by

    a. oral contraceptive use
    b. multiple pregnancies
    c. smoking
    d. none of the above

37–2. Prior to menopause, all of the following occur EXCEPT

    a. estradiol levels decrease
    b. inhibin levels increase
    c. progesterone levels decrease
    d. follicle-stimulating hormone (FSH) levels increase

37–3. Which of the following correctly describes estrogen in postmenopausal women?

    a. 17β-Estradiol is formed primarily by adrenal testosterone secretion.
    b. Estradiol levels exceed those of estrone.
    c. Obese women exhibit higher levels of estrogen than thin women.
    d. all of the above

37–4. What percentage of women will experience hot flashes in the first year of entering menopause (surgical or natural)?

    a. 50 percent
    b. 80 percent
    c. 90 percent
    d. 99 percent

37–5. Which of the following is the first event in the hot flash?

    a. increased muscular blood flow
    b. blood pressure increases
    c. cutaneous vasodilation
    d. none of the above

37–6. Which of the following hypoestrogenic states experiences hot flashes?

    a. gonadal dysgenesis
    b. premature ovarian failure
    c. hypothalamic failure
    d. all of the above

37–7. Which of the following is diagnostic of menopause?

    a. increased FSH levels
    b. low estradiol levels
    c. vaginal dryness
    d. all of the above

37–8. Which type or area of bone is highly sensitive to estrogen deficiency and/or replacement?

    a. trabecular
    b. thoracic vertebrae
    c. lumbar vertebrae
    d. all of the above

37–9. Which of the following increases the risk of osteoporosis?

    a. low high-density lipoprotein (HDL) levels
    b. heparin therapy
    c. hypothyroidism
    d. none of the above

37–10. Which of the following groups are NOT at high risk for development of osteoporosis?

    a. amenorrheic runners
    b. African-American men
    c. Oriental women
    d. none of the above

37–11. What percentage of women beyond the age of 80 will develop a hip fracture?

  a. 10 percent
  b. 25 percent
  c. 50 percent
  d. 80 percent

37–12. Which of the following locations and measurements of bone density is preferred?

  a. dual-energy x-ray absorptiometry (DEXA) of the hip
  b. computed tomography (CT) of the hip
  c. quantitative digital radiography (QDR) of the wrist
  d. sonography of the vertebral body

37–13. Which of the following is true regarding the incidence of age-matched mortality from cardiovascular disease?

  a. Men are at greater risk than women prior to menopause.
  b. Men are at less risk than women after menopause.
  c. Women are at greater risk than men at the time of menopause.
  d. all of the above

37–14. Treatment of men with estrogen

  a. reduces serum cholesterol levels
  b. reduces risk of death
  c. increases risk of colon cancer
  d. all of the above

37–15. Estrogen has which of the following actions?

  a. raises LDL
  b. lowers HDL
  c. raises very low-density lipoprotein (VLDL)
  d. all of the above

37–16. Which of the following regarding hot flashes is NOT true?

  a. blood flow decreases in muscle
  b. blood pressure rises
  c. blood flow increases in skin
  d. cutaneous vasodilation

37–17. During the hot flash, which of the following is true regarding LH pulses?

  a. Pulses of LH precede by 1 to 2 minutes the onset of the hot flash.
  b. LH pulses initiate the hot flash.
  c. Gonadotropin-releasing hormone (GnRH) agonists in postmenopausal women decrease LH and hot flashes.
  d. none of the above

37–18. Which of the following is true regarding norepinephrine?

  a. estrogen decreases synthesis
  b. binds to postjunctional receptors
  c. inhibits tyrosine hydroxylase
  d. monoamine oxidase stimulates synthesis

37–19. Estrogens have which of the following effects correlating to cognitive function?

  a. stimulate growth of cholinergic axons
  b. decrease acetylcholine
  c. decrease tyrosine hydroxylase
  d. stimulate amyloid deposition

37–20. Estrogens have which of the following effects on bone?

  a. decrease parathyroid hormone (PTH)
  b. decrease calcitonin
  c. increase urinary calcium
  d. bind to estrogen receptors on bone

37–21. Causes of secondary osteoporosis include

  a. glucocorticoids
  b. hyperthryoidism
  c. renal failure
  d. all of the above

37–22. Peak bone mass is achieved in women at what age?

  a. 20
  b. 30
  c. 40
  d. 50

37–23. Risk factors for osteoporosis include

  a. smoking
  b. alcohol

c. low body weight
d. all of the above

37–24. Vaginal atrophy is associated with all of the following EXCEPT

a. cell layer is 3 to 4 cells thick
b. vaginal walls are pale
c. cells contain more glycogen
d. reduced rugae

37–25. Which of the following hormone levels does NOT change following menopause?

a. estrone
b. androstenedione
c. cortisol
d. none of the above

37–26. Which of the following occurs following oophorectomy in postmenopausal women?

a. 17β-estradiol declines
b. testosterone declines
c. 17-OH progesterone decreases
d. all of the above

37–27. Which of the following is NOT true regarding lipids in postmenopausal women compared to age-matched men?

a. lower LDL
b. high HDL
c. similar VLDL levels
d. none of the above

Chapter 38

HORMONAL TREATMENT OF MENOPAUSAL WOMEN: RISKS AND BENEFITS

CASE REPORT

A 38-year-old white female, para 0-0-0-0, was evaluated for a second opinion regarding migraines and estrogen therapy relationship.

At age 26, the patient underwent a total abdominal hysterectomy and left salpingo-oophorectomy for a pelvic infection. Because of chronic pain, she had her right ovary removed at age 34. During the next 2 years, she took conjugated estrogens and micronized estradiol, and used the transdermal patch in an attempt to relieve migraine headaches. She had no complaints of hot flashes or vaginal dryness. She had been hospitalized four times with migraine headaches since age 34. In addition, she was taking meperidine (Demerol), diazepam (Valium), phenobarbital, and promethazine hydrochloride (Phenergan).

She had allergies to penicillin, phenytoin sodium (Dilantin), and sumatriptan succinate (Imitrex). There was no family history of migraines.

Magnetic resonance imaging (MRI) was negative. Numerous neurologists diagnosed her as status migraines or severe intractable migraines.

At age 36, she sought therapy from another physician who began treatment with estrogen pellets. Over the next 10 months, her physician implanted 34 estrogen pellets (25 mg), with occasional relief of migraines. The patient monitored her migraines but was unable to correlate with estrogen levels. The patient's estrogen levels were assayed at an outside assay using an extraction column technique. The normal upper limit in that assay for a menopausal woman was 13 pg/ml. The physician's goal was to reach an estradiol level of 50 to 100 pg/ml. The results of estradiol (E_2) assays by the outside lab and pellet insertion are seen in Figure 38–1. She complained of nausea, breast tenderness, and strange crawling sensations at the time she was evaluated at our institution. An assay at our laboratory using a standard immunoassay revealed estradiol levels >1000 pg/ml. No more pellets were given, and her estrogen levels fell slowly over the next year and were last measured to be 70 pg/ml. The patient was then started on a 0.1-mg estradiol patch. Remarkably, her headaches have significantly decreased, and presently she is doing well.

SUMMARY AND CONCLUSIONS

Although there is a correlation with estrogen deficiency and increased frequency of migraine headaches, if adequate "physiologic" levels of estrogen replacement are not effective, other medications and treatments regulated by neurologists are more appropriate. Estrogen replacement therapy (ERT) relieves hot flashes, vaginal dryness, insom-

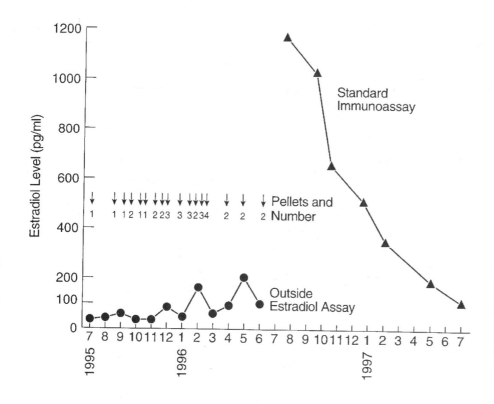

Figure 38–1. Relationship of estrogen pellet insertions (arrows) and number of pellets with two different assays for estradiol. The outside laboratory used an extraction and column technique with radioimmunoassay (RIA). The standard assay was Immulite®, chemiluminescent enzyme immunoassay *(Diagnostic Product Company, Los Angeles, CA).*

nia, and occasional headaches. Other benefits may include some relief from depression.

Monitoring estrogen levels in women on ERT and attempting to correlate levels with symptoms is not clinically useful and can be confusing, as noted in the present case. It is recommended that the standard estrogen assay be utilized, which is the same as that used to monitor follicular growth in infertility patients. Because of the interpretation of the assay illustrated in the present case, excessive numbers of pellets were inserted.

BIBLIOGRAPHY

Kudrow L. The relationship of headache frequency to hormone use in migraine. *Headache.* 15:36, 1975

Lichten EM, Lichten JB, Whitty AR, Pieper DM. The confirmation of a biochemical marker for women's hormonal migraine: the Depo-Estradiol challenge test. *Headache.* 36(6):367, 1996

Somerville BW. The role of estradiol withdrawal in the etiology of menstrual migraine. *Neurology.* 22:355, 1972

Stryker J. Use of hormones in women over 40. *Clin Obstet Gynecol.* 20(1):155, 1977

Welch KMA, Darnley D, Simkins RT. The role of estrogen in migraine: a review and hypothesis. *Cephalgia.* 4:227, 1984

QUESTIONS

38–1. ERT is associated with all of the following EXCEPT

   a. increased skin collagen
   b. decreased urinary incontinence
   c. increased weight gain
   d. decreased insomnia

38–2. Which of the following is the required daily dose of calcium for postmenopausal women?

   a. 500 mg
   b. 1000 mg
   c. 1500 mg
   d. 2000 mg

38–3. At what age does starting estrogen prevent further rapid loss of bone?

   a. 50
   b. 60
   c. 70
   d. all of the above

38–4. Which of the following treatments raises serum triglycerides?

    a. transdermal 17β-estradiol
    b. vaginal estrogen cream
    c. oral estrogen
    d. estrogen pellets

38–5. Which of the following is true regarding ERT?

    a. 50 percent reduction in cardiovascular disease
    b. reduction in subsequent myocardial infarctions
    c. reduction in coronary vessel low-density lipoprotein (LDL) incorporation
    d. all of the above

38–6. Which of the following is true regarding strokes?

    a. Estrogen plus progestins (hormone replacement therapy [HRT]) increase the risk of stroke.
    b. Estrogen (ERT) significantly reduces the risk of stroke.
    c. ERT significantly increases the risk of stroke.
    d. none of the above

38–7. Which of the following is true regarding Alzheimer's disease?

    a. It is more common in obese women.
    b. It is associated with high levels of acetylcholine.
    c. Estrogen delays the onset and severity of disease.
    d. all of the above

38–8. Estrogens alone without progestin (ERT) have all of the following effects in postmenopausal women EXCEPT

    a. decreased risk of ovarian cancer
    b. increased risk of endometrial cancer
    c. decreased risk of colon cancer
    d. slightly increased risk of breast cancer

38–9. Which of the following is correct regarding estrogen therapy in women with previous endometrial cancer?

    a. always contraindicated
    b. stage I, grade I, with minimal invasion; may treat immediately following surgery
    c. stage I, grade I, with minimal invasion; wait 5 years, then treat if no recurrence
    d. stage II always contraindicated

38–10. ERT is usually contraindicated in which of the following?

    a. previous pulmonary embolus
    b. gallbladder disease
    c. diabetes mellitus
    d. all of the above

38–11. When is an endometrial biopsy indicated in ERT users?

    a. bleeding heavily prior to therapy
    b. endometrial thickness is 7 mm
    c. women on estrogen therapy alone
    d. all of the above

38–12. Tamoxifen has all of the following characteristics and actions EXCEPT

    a. it increases bone content
    b. estrogenic effects
    c. it increases endometrial hyperplasia
    d. it reduces hot flashes

38–13. Alendronate has which of the following effects?

    a. well absorbed orally
    b. useful for treatment of osteomalacia
    c. can cause brittle bones
    d. can cause esophagitis

38–14. Which of the following is correct in women using ERT/HRT?

    a. Use >10 years may increase the risk of breast cancer.
    b. Use <5 years increases the risk of breast cancer.
    c. The death rate from breast cancer is greater in ERT users than in nonusers.
    d. all of the above

38–15. Alternative therapies for estrogen to treat vasomotor symptoms include

   a. progestins
   b. vitamin E
   c. diazepam (Valium)
   d. all of the above

38–16. Which of the following is true regarding the minimal estrogen dose and prevention of fractures in the hip?

   a. Premarin, 1.25 mg
   b. Ogen, 1.25 mg
   c. Estrace, 0.5 mg
   d. Premarin, 0.3 mg

38–17. Tacrine is a drug used to treat which of the following?

   a. cataracts
   b. osteoporosis
   c. Alzheimer's disease
   d. ovarian cancer

38–18. Meta-analysis of studies of stress urinary incontinence suggest that

   a. incidence increases with age
   b. estrogen has little effect
   c. adrenergic agents plus estrogen are more effective than estrogen alone
   d. all of the above

38–19. Weight gain in postmenopausal women is due to

   a. combined HRT
   b. aging
   c. an estrogen component
   d. a progestin component

38–20. Routine screening bone densities are not measured in all women because of

   a. radiation exposure
   b. the length of the procedure
   c. the cost
   d. all of the above

38–21. In women with cardiovascular disease, estrogens have all of the following effects EXCEPT

   a. they decrease risk of myocardial infarction (MI)
   b. they decrease coronary occlusion on arteriograms
   c. they are always contraindicated
   d. none of the above

38–22. In women who smoke

   a. the risk of MI is greater in ERT users than in nonusers
   b. estrogen levels are more increased in ERT users than in nonsmoking ERT users
   c. and use ERT, they are at increased risk for cervical cancer than in non-ERT users
   d. none of the above

38–23. In comparing rates of death in women with endometrial cancer, which of the following is true?

   a. similar in ERT users versus nonusers
   b. significantly decreased in users of ERT compared to nonusers
   c. significantly increased in previous users of ERT compared to nonusers
   d. slightly increased in HRT users versus nonusers

38–24. The development of gallstones is associated with or due to which of the following?

   a. Studies show lower risk in oral versus transdermal estrogen usage.
   b. They are a common complication of HRT.
   c. They are more common in women than in men.
   d. all of the above

38–25. Which of the following is true regarding androstenedione?

   a. converted to estrogen in fat
   b. increased levels found in post-menopausal women compared to pre-menopausal women
   c. increases triglycerides
   d. all of the above

38–26. Estrogen is contraindicated in

    a. hypertension
    b. ovarian cancer
    c. both of the above
    d. none of the above

38–27. Which of the following disorders occurs last in postmenopausal women?

    a. vaginal dryness
    b. Alzheimer's disease
    c. osteoporosis
    d. cardiovascular disease

ANSWERS

CHAPTER 1

1–1. c *(p. 1)*

1–2. d *(p. 2)*

1–3. c *(p. 1)*

1–4. b *(p. 3)*

1–5. a *(p. 4)*

1–6. c *(p. 6)*

1–7. c *(p. 9)*

1–8. d *(p. 9)*

1–9. d *(p. 6)*

1–10. b *(p. 9)*

1–11. d *(p. 10)*

1–12. d *(p. 10)*

1–13. b *(p. 10)*

1–14. b *(p. 9)*

1–15. c *(p. 3)*

1–16. a *(p. 2)*

1–17. b *(p. 3)*

1–18. b *(p. 5)*

1–19. c *(p. 4)*

1–20. d *(p. 8)*

1–21. b *(p. 9)*

1–22. c *(p. 11)*

1–23. d *(p. 10)*

1–24. c *(p. 10)*

1–25. d *(p. 10)*

1–26. d *(p. 8)*

1–27. b *(p. 3)*

CHAPTER 2

2–1. a *(p. 19)*

2–2. c *(p. 19)*

2–3. a *(p. 21)*

2–4. a *(p. 22)*

2–5. a *(p. 22)*

2–6. c *(p. 23)*

2–7. b *(p. 24)*

2–8. d *(p. 24)*

2–9. d *(p. 24)*

2–10. c *(p. 27)*

2–11. d *(p. 28)*

2–12. b *(p. 31)*

2–13. c *(p. 31)*

2–14. a *(p. 32)*

2–15. c (*p. 34*)

2–16. b (*p. 20*)

2–17. d (*p. 22*)

2–18. b (*p. 21*)

2–19. d (*p. 26*)

2–20. d (*p. 27*)

2–21. c (*p. 28*)

2–22. c (*p. 32*)

2–23. d (*p. 24*)

2–24. a (*p. 25*)

2–25. c (*p. 25*)

2–26. c (*p. 28*)

2–27. c (*p. 30*)

CHAPTER 3

3–1. a (*p. 45*)

3–2. c (*p. 45*)

3–3. d (*p. 47*)

3–4. c (*p. 48*)

3–5. d (*p. 49*)

3–6. a (*p. 49*)

3–7. a (*p. 49*)

3–8. c (*p. 49*)

3–9. a (*p. 50*)

3–10. d (*p. 53*)

3–11. a (*p. 53*)

3–12. b (*p. 53*)

3–13. b (*p. 52*)

3–14. b (*p. 52*)

3–15. d (*p. 48*)

3–16. d (*p. 47*)

3–17. a (*p. 45*)

3–18. c (*p. 47*)

3–19. c (*p. 47*)

3–20. c (*p. 48*)

3–21. d (*p. 48*)

3–22. b (*p. 49*)

3–23. a (*p. 50*)

3–24. b (*p. 51*)

3–25. d (*p. 52*)

3–26. d (*p. 53*)

3–27. a (*p. 52*)

CHAPTER 4

4–1. b (*p. 57*)

4–2. d (*p. 58*)

4–3. b (*p. 58*)

4–4. a (*p. 60*)

4–5. b (*p. 61*)

4–6. d (*p. 62*)

4–7. d (*p. 62*)

4–8. d (*p. 64*)

4–9. b (*p. 66*)

4–10. c (*p. 68*)

4–11. c (*p. 69*)

4–12. d (*p. 70*)

4–13. c (*p. 74*)

4–14. a (*p. 76*)

4–15. a (*p. 76*)

4–16. a (*p. 78*)

4–17. d (*p. 79*)

4–18. b (*p. 80*)

4–19. c (*p. 84*)

4–20. c (*p. 87*)

4–21. a (*p. 57*)

4–22. c (*p. 58*)

4–23. c (*p. 58*)

4–24. c (*p. 67*)

4–25. b (*p. 67*)

4–26. c (*p. 62*)

4–27. c (*p. 81*)

4–28. d (*p. 81*)

4–29. d (*p. 83*)

4–30. d (*p. 86*)

4–31. d (*p. 87*)

4–32. a (*p. 84*)

CHAPTER 5

5–1. b (*p. 94*)

5–2. c (*p.94*)

5–3. b (*p. 94*)

5–4. c (*p. 95*)

5–5. c (*p. 95*)

5–6. c (*p. 96*)

5–7. b (*p. 96*)

5–8. c (*p. 100*)

5–9. b (*p. 100*)

5–10. d (*p. 102*)

5–11. b (*p. 104*)

5–12. d (*p. 104*)

5–13. b (*p. 106*)

5–14. b (*p. 108*)

5–15. b (*p. 107*)

5–16. a (*p. 96*)

5–17. b (*p. 93*)

5–18. b (*p. 94*)

5–19. d (*p. 95*)

5–20. b (*p. 95*)

5–21. b (*p. 97*)

5–22. d (*p. 98*)

5–23. c (*p. 99*)

5–24. b (*p. 99*)

5–25. d (*p. 99*)

5–26. c (*p. 99*)

5–27. b (*p. 108*)

CHAPTER 6

6–1. b (*p. 117*)

6–2. a (*p. 114*)

6–3. c (*p. 114*)

6–4. d (*p. 115*)

6–5. d (*p. 116*)

6–6. c (*p. 116*)

6–7. b (*p. 116*)

6–8. b (*p. 118*)

6–9. d (*p. 117*)

6–10. b (*p. 118*)

6–11. a (*p. 119*)

6–12. b (*p. 122*)

6–13. b (*p. 122*)

6–14. d (*p. 124*)

6–15. b (*p. 126*)

6–16. b (*p. 129*)

6–17. b (*p. 129*)

6–18. d (*p. 130*)

6–19. d (*p. 131*)

6–20. c (*p. 124*)

6–21. b (*p. 114*)

6–22. b (*p. 114*)

6–23. d (*p. 117*)

6–24. c (*p. 116*)

6–25. d (*p. 117*)

6–26. d (*p. 119*)

6–27. d (*p. 119*)

6–28. d (*p. 121*)

6–29. b (*p. 125*)

6–30. b (*p. 126*)

CHAPTER 7

7–1. c (*p. 137*)

7–2. a (*p. 137*)

7–3. d (*p. 138*)

7–4. a (*p. 138*)

7–5. d (*p. 138*)

7–6. b (*p. 139*)

7–7. d (*p. 139*)

7–8. c (*p. 141*)

7–9. b (*p. 142*)

7–10. c (*p. 143*)

7–11. b (*p. 144*)

7–12. d (*p. 145*)

7–13. b (*p. 148*)

7–14. a (*p. 148*)

7–15. d (*p. 153*)

7–16. d (*p. 137*)

7–17. b (*p. 137*)

7–18. b (*p. 138*)

7–19. c (*p. 138*)

7–20. d (*p. 138*)

7–21. c (*p. 139*)

7–22. c (*p. 143*)

7–23. d (*p. 146*)

7–24. c (*p. 140*)

7–25. b (*p. 141*)

7–26. c (*p. 142*)

7–27. c (*p. 143*)

CHAPTER 8

8–1. b (*p. 157*)

8–2. d (*p. 157*)

8–3. c (*p. 157*)

8–4. b (*p. 162*)

8–5. c (*p. 158*)

8–6. d (*p. 158*)

8–7. c (*p. 166*)

8–8. d (*p. 158*)

8–9. a (*p. 164*)

8–10. d (*p. 160*)

8–11. d (*p. 160*)

8–12. c (*p. 161*)

8–13. d (*p. 162*)

8–14. d (*p. 163*)

8–15. d (*p. 164*)

8–16. a (*p. 157*)

8–17. d (*p. 159*)

8–18. d (*p. 163*)

8–19. d (*p. 159*)

8–20. a (*p. 159*)

8–21. c (*p. 160*)

8–22. c (*p. 161*)

8–23. d (*p. 161*)

8–24. d (*p. 161*)

8–25. a (*p. 160*)

8–26. b (*p. 160*)

8–27. d (*p. 162*)

CHAPTER 9

9–1. d (*p. 174*)

9–2. b (*p. 173*)

9–3. a (*p. 173*)

9–4. b (*p. 292*)

9–5. d (*p. 173*)

9–6. a (*p. 173*)

9–7. c (*p. 174*)

9–8. c (*p. 174*)

9–9. c (*p. 175*)

9–10. c (*p. 175*)

9–11. a (*p. 175*)

9–12. d (*p. 176*)

9–13. d (*p. 176*)

9–14. c (*p. 181*)

9–15. d (*p. 181*)

9–16. c (*p. 184*)

9–17. c (*p. 185*)

9–18. d (*p. 173*)

9–19. a (*p. 173*)

9–20. a (*p. 173*)

9–21. c (*p. 173*)

9–22. a (*p. 177*)

9–23. d (*p. 176*)

9–24. d (*p. 178*)

9–25. c (*p. 178*)

9–26. d (*p. 180*)

9–27. b (*p. 180*)

9–28. a (*p. 178*)

9–29. d (*p. 183*)

CHAPTER 10

10–1. d (*p. 200*)

10–2. d (*p. 201*)

10–3. c (*p. 193*)

10–4. c (*p. 199*)

10–5. d (*p. 194*)

10–6. c (*p. 199*)

10–7. d (*p. 194*)

10–8. c (*p. 195*)

10–9. b (*p. 195*)

10–10. a (*p. 196*)

10–11. d (*p. 196*)

10–12. d (*p. 199*)

10–13. d (*p. 200*)

10–14. b (*p. 201*)

10–15. a (*p. 193*)

10–16. b (*p. 196*)

10–17. d (*p. 199*)

10–18. a (*p. 200*)

10–19. c (*p. 201*)

10–20. b (*p. 194*)

10–21. c (*p. 194*)

10–22. c (*p. 195*)

10–23. b (*p. 194*)

10–24. a (*p. 195*)

10–25. c (*p. 195*)

10–26. d (*p. 196*)

CHAPTER 11

11–1. b (*p. 207*)

11–2. d (*p. 207*)

11–3. c (*p. 208*)

11–4. d (*p. 209*)

11–5. b (*p. 209*)

11–6. c (*p. 211*)

11–7. a (*p. 214*)

11–8. c (*p. 216*)

11–9. c (*p. 214*)

11–10. c (*p. 215*)

11–11. a (*p. 215*)

11–12. b (*p. 216*)

11–13. a (*p. 216*)

11–14. c (*p. 217*)

11–15. d (*p. 217*)

11–16. d (*p. 219*)

11–17. d (*p. 219*)

11–18. a (*p. 219*)

11–19. b (*p. 219*)

11–20. a (*p. 223*)

11–21. b (*p. 207*)

11–22. c (*p. 208*)

11–23. b (*p. 211*)

11–24. b (*p. 210*)

11–25. c (*p. 210*)

11–26. d (*p. 211*)

11–27. a (*p. 211*)

11–28. c (*p. 211*)

11–29. d (*p. 225*)

11–30. a (*p. 217*)

11–31. d (*p. 220*)

11–32. d (*p. 222*)

CHAPTER 12

12–1. b (*p. 233*)

12–2. d (*p. 233*)

12–3. c (*p. 233*)

12–4. d (*p. 233*)

12–5. d (*p. 234*)

12–6. c (*p. 234*)

12–7. c (*p. 234*)

12–8. b (*p. 235*)

12–9. d (*p. 235*)

12–10. d (*p. 236*)

12–11. b (*p. 236*)

12–12. a (*p. 236*)

12–13. b (*p. 236*)

12–14. c (*p. 237*)

12–15. d (*p. 240*)

12–16. d (*p. 233*)

12–17. b (*p. 233*)

12–18. c (*p. 234*)

12–19. d (*p. 235*)

12–20. c (*p. 236*)

12–21. a (*p. 236*)

12–22. c (*p. 236*)

12–23. d (*p. 236*)

12–24. a (*p. 236*)

12–25. c (*p. 237*)

12–26. d (*p. 238*)

12–27. c (*p. 238*)

CHAPTER 13

13–1. b (*p. 245*)

13–2. c (*p. 248*)

13–3. d (*p. 248*)

13–4. d (*p. 249*)

13–5. b (*p. 249*)

13–6. d (*p. 252*)

13–7. d (*p. 251*)

13–8. c (*p. 251*)

13–9. c (*p. 252*)

13–10. c (*p. 252*)

13–11. c (*p. 254*)

13–12. a (*p. 254*)

13–13. c (*p. 263*)

13–14. d (*p. 255*)

13–15. c (*p. 256*)

13–16. b (*p. 256*)

13–17. b (*p. 257*)

13–18. b (*p. 257*)

13–19. a (*p. 258*)

13–20. b (*p. 259*)

13–21. c (*p. 259*)

13–22. d (*p. 260*)

13–23. c (*p. 245*)

13–24. b (*p. 245*)

13–25. d (*p. 246*)

13–26. a (*p. 246*)

13–27. c (*p. 246*)

13–28. c (*p. 248*)

13–29. b (*p. 257*)

13–30. a (*p. 258*)

13–31. d (*p. 261*)

13–32. c (*p. 246*)

CHAPTER 14

14–1. d (*p. 271*)

14–2. d (*p. 272*)

14–3. d (*p. 272*)

14–4. c (*p. 273*)

14–5. c (*p. 273*)

14–6. c (*p. 274*)

14–7. c (*p. 274*)

14–8. b (*p. 276*)

14–9. c (*p. 277*)

14–10. d (*p. 277*)

14–11. b (*p. 278*)

14–12. d (*p. 279*)

14–13. b (*p. 279*)

14–14. d (*p. 284*)

14–15. c (*p. 279*)

14–16. c (*p. 274*)

14–17. c (*p. 276*)

14–18. c (*p. 281*)

14–19. b (*p. 280*)

14–20. d (*p. 280*)

14–21. a (*p. 281*)

14–22. d (*p. 281*)

14–23. d (*p. 284*)

14–24. c (*p. 279*)

14–25. b (*p. 279*)

14–26. c (*p. 281*)

14–27. c (*p. 279*)

CHAPTER 15

15–1. d (*p. 292*)

15–2. d (*p. 303*)

15–3. d (*p. 303*)

15–4. c (*p. 295*)

15–5. c (*p. 290*)

15–6. a (*p. 289*)

15–7. c (*p. 292*)

15–8. c (*p. 293*)

15–9. b (*p. 294*)

15–10. d (*p. 297*)

15–11. d (*p. 298*)

15–12. d (*p. 302*)

15–13. b (*p. 301*)

15–14. c (*p. 302*)

15–15. d (*p. 289*)

15–16. b (*p. 295*)

15–17. d (*p. 290*)

15–18. c (*p. 289*)

15–19. c (*p. 302*)

15–20. d (*p. 298*)

15–21. d (*p. 296*)

15–22. a (*p. 295*)

15–23. d (*p. 295*)

15–24. d (*p. 301*)

15–25. d (*p. 301*)

15–26. c (*p. 302*)

CHAPTER 16

16–1. d (*p. 309*)

16–2. c (*p. 315*)

16–3. a (*p. 315*)

16–4. d (*p. 314*)

16–5. c (*p. 311*)

16–6. a (*p. 309*)

16–7. d (*p. 312*)

16–8. b (*p. 313*)

16–9. c (*p. 313*)

16–10. d (*p. 313*)

16–11. c (*p. 314*)

16–12. d (*p. 314*)

16–13. c (*p. 315*)

16–14. a (*p. 315*)

16–15. d (*p. 316*)

16–16. a (*p. 309*)

16–17. d (*p. 312*)

16–18. a (*p. 309*)

16–19. b (*p. 313*)

16–20. d (*p. 314*)

16–21. a (*p. 315*)

16–22. d (*p. 317*)

16–23. d (*p. 313*)

16–24. d (*p. 317*)

16–25. b (*p. 317*)

16–26. b (*p. 317*)

CHAPTER 17

17–1. d (*p. 323*)

17–2. b (*p. 323*)

17–3. d (*p. 325*)

17–4. d (*p. 327*)

17–5. d (*p. 328*)

17–6. a (*p. 328*)

17–7. d (*p. 329*)

17–8. b (*p. 329*)

17–9. d (*p. 331*)

17–10. b (*p. 331*)

17–11. d (*p. 333*)

17–12. c (*p. 334*)

17–13. d (*p. 334*)

17–14. d (*p. 334*)

17–15. c (*p. 335*)

17–16. d (*p. 335*)

17–17. d (*p. 337*)

17–18. d (*p. 343*)

17–19. d (*p. 323*)

17–20. c (*p. 324*)

17–21. d (*p. 325*)

17–22. a (*p. 325*)

17–23. d (*p. 324*)

17–24. b (*p. 326*)

17–25. d (*p. 327*)

17–26. d (*p. 324*)

17–27. d (*p. 335*)

CHAPTER 18

18–1. b (*p. 353*)

18–2. d (*p. 376*)

18–3. a (*p. 354*)

18–4. d (*p. 355*)

18–5. d (*p. 355*)

18–6. b (*p. 356*)

18–7. b (*p. 359*)

18–8. d (*p. 360*)

18–9. c (*p. 374*)

18–10. d (*p. 362*)

18–11. d (*p. 366*)

18–12. c (*p. 368*)

18–13. d (*p. 369*)

18–14. c (*p. 373*)

18–15. a (*p. 375*)

18–16. c (*p. 375*)

18–17. b (*p. 375*)

18–18. d (*p. 353*)

18–19. d (*p. 352*)

18–20. d (*p. 354*)

18–21. d (*p. 355*)

18–22. d (*p. 355*)

18–23. a (*p. 356*)

18–24. a (*p. 356*)

18–25. c (*p. 356*)

18–26. b (*p. 357*)

18–27. d (*p. 359*)

19–14. d (*p. 399*)

19–15. d (*p. 400*)

19–16. d (*p. 400*)

19–17. d (*p. 395*)

19–18. d (*p. 393*)

19–20. d (*p. 393*)

19–21. c (*p. 396*)

19–22. c (*p. 392*)

19–23. d (*p. 395*)

19–24. a (*p. 395*)

19–25. d (*p. 396*)

19–26. a (*p. 395*)

CHAPTER 19

19–1. d (*p. 389*)

19–2. a (*p. 389*)

19–3. d (*p. 390*)

19–4. d (*p. 392*)

19–5. d (*p. 393*)

19–6. d (*p. 393*)

19–7. d (*p. 395*)

19–8. d (*p. 395*)

19–9. d (*p. 395*)

19–10. c (*p. 395*)

19–11. c (*p. 396*)

19–12. d (*p. 398*)

19–13. c (*p. 399*)

CHAPTER 20

20–1. d (*p. 405*)

20–2. d (*p. 406*)

20–3. a (*p. 408*)

20–4. c (*p. 408*)

20–5. b (*p. 409*)

20–6. c (*p. 411*)

20–7. a (*p. 411*)

20–8. d (*p. 412*)

20–9. d (*p. 413*)

20–10. c (*p. 412*)

20–11. d (*p. 414*)

20–12. b (*p. 418*)

20–13. c (*p. 420*)

20–14. d (*p. 419*)

20–15. d (*p. 416*)

20–16. c (*p. 413*)

20–17. c (*p. 405*)

20–18. c (*p. 409*)

20–19. a (*p. 412*)

20–20. c (*p. 407*)

20–21. d (*p. 409*)

20–22. a (*p. 411*)

20–23. d (*p. 411*)

20–24. b (*p. 412*)

20–25. c (*p. 412*)

20–26. d (*p. 412*)

20–27. a (*p. 417*)

CHAPTER 21

21–1. d (*p. 425*)

21–2. b (*p. 426*)

21–3. a (*p. 427*)

21–4. d (*p. 429*)

21–5. b (*p. 430*)

21–6. d (*p. 430*)

21–7. d (*p. 435*)

21–8. a (*p. 434*)

21–9. b (*p. 433*)

21–10. c (*p. 435*)

21–11. c (*p. 443*)

21–12. b (*p. 437*)

21–13. d (*p. 438*)

21–14. b (*p. 440*)

21–15. a (*p. 441*)

21–16. d (*p. 429*)

21–17. b (*p. 430*)

21–18. a (*p. 441*)

21–19. a (*p. 442*)

21–20. b (*p. 442*)

21–21. a (*p. 437*)

21–22. b (*p. 435*)

21–23. b (*p. 434*)

21–24. c (*p. 434*)

21–25. d (*p. 430*)

21–26. c (*p. 434*)

21–27. b (*p. 433*)

CHAPTER 22

22–1. c (*p. 455*)

22–2. d (*p. 455*)

22–3. b (*p. 457*)

22–4. d (*p. 459*)

22–5. b (*p. 458*)

22–6. b (*p. 459*)

22–7. c (*p. 459*)

22–8. d (*p. 461*)

22–9. d (*p. 461*)

22–10. d (*p. 462*)

22–11. a (*p. 463*)

22–12. d (*p. 463*)

22–13. d (*p. 462*)

22–14. b (*p. 462*)

22–15. d (*p. 459*)

22–16. d (*p. 457*)

22–17. a (*p. 455*)

22–18. d (*p. 455*)

22–19. b (*p. 455*)

22–20. d (*p. 455*)

22–21. d (*p. 455*)

22–22. c (*p. 456*)

22–23. d (*p. 456*)

22–24. a (*p. 457*)

22–25. d (*p. 457*)

22–26. d (*p. 457*)

CHAPTER 23

23–1. c (*p. 467*)

23–2. d (*p. 467*)

23–3. b (*p. 470*)

23–4. d (*p. 468*)

23–5. c (*p. 469*)

23–6. b (*p. 469*)

23–7. c (*p. 473*)

23–8. d (*p. 471*)

23–9. b (*p. 472*)

23–10. c (*p. 474*)

23–11. d (*p. 471*)

23–12. d (*p. 477*)

23–13. a (*p. 477*)

23–14. c (*p. 478*)

23–15. a (*p. 479*)

23–16. d (*p. 473*)

23–17. c (*p. 467*)

23–18. b (*p. 467*)

23–19. a (*p. 468*)

23–20. c (*p. 468*)

23–21. d (*p. 469*)

23–22. d (*p. 469*)

23–23. c (*p. 471*)

23–24. d (*p. 472*)

23–25. c (*p. 473*)

23–26. d (*p. 472*)

23–27. c (*p. 478*)

CHAPTER 24

24–1. d (*p. 491*)

24–2. d (*p. 492*)

24–3. d (*p. 492*)

24–4. c (*p. 492*)

24–5. d (*p. 485*)

24–6. c (*p. 486*)

24–7. d (*p. 485*)

24–8. d (*p. 486*)

24–9. d (*p. 486*)

24–10. c (*p. 486*)

24–11. a (*p. 486*)

24–12. c (*p. 489*)

24–13. d (*p. 490*)

24–14. d (*p. 489*)

24–15. d (*p. 490*)

24–16. d (*p. 490*)

24–17. d (*p. 489*)

24–18. a (*p. 490*)

24–19. a (*p. 489*)

24–20. d (*p. 489*)

24–21. d (*p. 489*)

24–22. a (*p. 489*)

24–23. d (*p. 489*)

24–24. d (*p. 489*)

24–25. d (*p. 489*)

24–26. d (*p. 490*)

CHAPTER 25

25–1. b (*p. 496*)

25–2. d (*p. 496*)

25–3. b (*p. 498*)

25–4. a (*p. 499*)

25–5. d (*p. 500*)

25–6. a (*p. 501*)

25–7. a (*p. 502*)

25–8. d (*p. 503*)

25–9. c (*p. 503*)

25–10. c (*p. 503*)

25–11. a (*p. 503*)

25–12. d (*p. 504*)

25–13. c (*p. 505*)

25–14. d (*p. 511*)

25–15. d (*p. 512*)

25–16. a (*p. 495*)

25–17. c (*p. 495*)

25–18. d (*p. 495*)

25–19. a (*p. 496*)

25–20. b (*p. 496*)

25–21. d (*p. 497*)

25–22. b (*p. 497*)

25–23. a (*p. 506*)

25–24. c (*p. 499*)

25–25. b (*p. 500*)

25–26. d (*p. 503*)

25–27. a (*p. 511*)

CHAPTER 26

26–1. d (*p. 520*)

26–2. d (*p. 520*)

26–3. d (*p. 531*)

26–4. d (*p. 521*)

26–5. c (*p. 521*)

26–6. b (*p. 522*)

26–7. d (*p. 523*)

26–8. d (*p. 523*)

26–9. d (*p. 523*)

26–10. d (*p. 523*)

26–11. d (*p. 530*)

26–12. a (*p. 523*)

26–13. d (*p. 526*)

26–14. b (*p. 521*)

26–15. d (*p. 520*)

26–16. d (*p. 518*)

26–17. d (*p. 519*)

26–18. a (*p. 517*)

26–19. d (*p. 518*)

26–20. d (*p. 518*)

26–21. d (*p. 519*)

26–22. b (*p. 519*)

26–23. c (*p. 519*)

26–24. b (*p. 519*)

26–25. d (*p. 520*)

26–26. d (*p. 520*)

CHAPTER 27

27–1. a (*p. 534*)

27–2. c (*p. 534*)

27–3. d (*p. 535*)

27–4. c (*p. 535*)

27–5. a (*p. 537*)

27–6. a (*p. 538*)

27–7. c (*p. 539*)

27–8. b (*p. 542*)

27–9. b (*p. 541*)

27–10. c (*p. 542*)

27–11. c (*p. 542*)

27–12. c (*p. 544*)

27–13. d (*p. 545*)

27–14. c (*p. 539*)

27–15. b (*p. 544*)

27–16. a (*p. 541*)

27–17. a (*p. 541*)

27–18. b (*p. 539*)

27–19. d (*p. 543*)

27–20. c (*p. 544*)

27–21. c (*p. 544*)

27–22. d (*p. 544*)

27–23. c (*p. 538*)

27–24. d (*p. 541*)

27–25. d (*p. 540*)

27–26. d (*p. 542*)

27–27. a (*p. 543*)

CHAPTER 28

28–1. b (*p. 549*)

28–2. c (*p. 549*)

28–3. a (*p. 550*)

28–4. d (*p. 551*)

28–5. d (*p. 551*)

28–6. a (*p. 551*)

28–7. b (*p. 551*)

28–8. a (*p. 551*)

28–9. c (*p. 552*)

28–10. d (*p. 553*)

28–11. d (*p. 554*)

28–12. d (*p. 554*)

28–13. d (*p. 555*)

28–14. d (*p. 559*)

28–15. d (*p. 559*)

28–16. c (*p. 549*)

28–17. b (*p. 551*)

28–18. c (*p. 558*)

28–19. c (*p. 559*)

28–20. b (*p. 550*)

28–21. d (*p. 550*)

28–22. d (*p. 551*)

28–23. a (*p. 551*)

28–24. b (*p. 552*)

28–25. c (*p. 553*)

28–26. b (*p. 554*)

28–27. d (*p. 555*)

CHAPTER 29

29–1. a (*p. 565*)

29–2. d (*p. 565*)

29–3. c (*p. 566*)

29–4. d (*p. 566*)

29–5. d (*p. 566*)

29–6. c (*p. 567*)

29–7. d (*p. 567*)

29–8. a (*p. 568*)

29–9. c (*p. 568*)

29–10. d (*p. 569*)

29–11. b (*p. 577*)

29–12. c (*p. 568*)

29–13. b (*p. 577*)

29–14. d (*p. 577*)

29–15. b (*p. 565*)

29–16. d (*p. 565*)

29–17. d (*p. 568*)

29–18. c (*p. 567*)

29–19. d (*p. 567*)

29–20. c (*p. 567*)

29–21. d (*p. 567*)

29–22. d (*p. 568*)

29–23. d (*p. 568*)

29–24. d (*p. 565*)

29–25. c (*p. 568*)

29–26. d (*p. 571*)

29–27. c (*p. 571*)

29–28. c (*p. 568*)

CHAPTER 30

30–1. b (*p. 583*)

30–2. d (*p. 587*)

30–3. a (*p. 587*)

30–4. c (*p. 590*)

30–5. b (*p. 593*)

30–6. b (*p. 594*)

30–7. a (*p. 595*)

30–8. b (*p. 597*)

30–9. a (*p. 597*)

30–10. d (*p. 596*)

30–11. d (*p. 597*)

30–12. b (*p. 599*)

30–13. b (*p. 600*)

30–14. c (*p. 600*)

30–15. b (*p. 603*)

30–16. d (*p. 585*)

30–17. d (*p. 587*)

30–18. c (*p. 589*)

30–19. d (*p. 591*)

30–20. c (*p. 597*)

30–21. b (*p. 590*)

30–22. c (*p. 592*)

30–23. b (*p. 598*)

30–24. d (*p. 598*)

30–25. c (*p. 598*)

30–26. d (*p. 600*)

30–27. c (*p. 601*)

CHAPTER 31

31–1. b (*p. 607*)

31–2. b (*p. 607*)

31–3. d (*p. 607*)

31–4. b (*p. 608*)

31–5. d (*p. 609*)

31–6. c (*p. 609*)

31–7. d (*p. 609*)

31–8. c (*p. 609*)

31–9. d (*p. 610*)

31–10. d (*p. 610*)

31–11. d (*p. 609*)

31–12. b (*p. 611*)

31–13. d (*p. 611*)

31–14. c (*p. 613*)

31–15. a (*p. 618*)

31–16. d (*p. 617*)

31–17. a (*p. 617*)

31–18. c (*p. 617*)

31–19. c (*p. 617*)

31–20. b (*p. 622*)

31–21. d (*p. 613*)

31–22. d (*p. 612*)

31–23. c (*p. 613*)

31–24. c (*p. 615*)

31–25. a (*p. 611*)

31–26. d (*p. 618*)

31–27. b (*p. 622*)

CHAPTER 32

32–1. a (*p. 644*)

32–2. d (*p. 642*)

32–3. a (*p. 644*)

32–4. d (*p. 644*)

32–5. c (*p. 646*)

32–6. d (*p. 646*)

32–7. c (*p. 647*)

32–8. c (*p. 648*)

32–9. d (*p. 650*)

32–10. b (*p. 650*)

32–11. d (*p. 651*)

32–12. b (*p. 652*)

32–13. d (*p. 652*)

32–14. b (*p. 654*)

32–15. a (*p. 658*)

32–16. d (*p. 641*)

32–17. d (*p. 642*)

32–18. c (*p. 646*)

32–19. b (*p. 646*)

32–20. c (*p. 649*)

32–21. d (*p. 645*)

32–22. c (*p. 647*)

32–23. a (*p. 648*)

32–24. c (*p. 650*)

32–25. c (*p. 650*)

32–26. a (*p. 650*)

32–27. d (*p. 655*)

CHAPTER 33

33–1. b (*p. 610*)

33–2. c (*p. 665*)

33–3. c (*p. 666*)

33–4. d (*p. 666*)

33–5. d (*p. 665*)

33–6. c (*p. 665*)

33–7. c (*p. 666*)

33–8. c (*p. 666*)

33–9. c (*p. 666*)

33–10. d (*p. 667*)

33–11. d (*p. 667*)

33–12. d (*p. 668*)

33–13. d (*p. 668*)

33–14. d (*p. 669*)

33–15. c (*p. 665*)

33–16. c (*p. 666*)

33–17. a (*p. 666*)

33–18. d (*p. 667*)

33–19. d (*p. 667*)

33–20. c (*p. 667*)

33–21. b (*p. 667*)

33–22. c (*p. 668*)

33–23. b (*p. 667*)

33–24. b (*p. 669*)

33–25. d (*p. 670*)

33–26. c (*p. 672*)

33–27. d (*p. 672*)

CHAPTER 34

34–1. d (*p. 679*)

34–2. b (*p. 679*)

34–3. b (*p. 679*)

34–4. d (*p. 680*)

34–5. b (*p. 680*)

34–6. c (*p. 681*)

34–7. a (*p. 681*)

34–8. a (*p. 682*)

34–9. a (*p. 683*)

34–10. ~~(p. 683)~~ *or C*

34–11. c (*p. 684*)

34–12. d (*p. 686*)

34–13. a (*p. 686*)

34–14. a (*p. 688*)

34–15. a (*p. 680*)

34–16. b (*p. 681*)

34–17. d (*p. 681*)

34–18. b (*p. 681*)

34–19. d (*p. 682*)

34–20. b (*p. 682*)

34–21. c (*p. 682*)

34–22. c (*p. 682*)

34–23. c (*p. 685*)

34–24. a (*p. 683*)

34–25. b (*p. 685*)

34–26. d (*p. 683*)

34–27. d (*p. 683*)

CHAPTER 35

35–1. d (*p. 694*)

35–2. d (*p. 698*)

35–3. d (*p. 693*)

35–4. d (*p. 693*)

35–5. c (*p. 694*)

35–6. d (*p. 694*)

35–7. d (*p. 696*)

35–8. c (*p. 694*)

35–9. c (*p. 694*)

35–10. d (*p. 695*)

35–11. d (*p. 697*)

35–12. b (*p. 698*)

35–13. d (*p. 697*)

35–14. a (*p. 701*)

35–15. d (*p. 703*)

CHAPTER 36

36–1. b *(p. 707)*

36–2. a *(p. 710)*

36–3. b *(p. 711)*

36–4. c *(p. 711)*

36–5. d *(p. 711)*

36–6. c *(p. 712)*

36–7. d *(p. 712)*

36–8. c *(p. 712)*

36–9. b *(p. 713)*

36–10. d *(p. 715)*

36–11. a *(p. 717)*

36–12. b *(p. 715)*

36–13. d *(p. 719)*

36–14. b *(p. 720)*

36–15. a *(p. 721)*

36–16. d *(p. 707)*

36–17. c *(p. 708)*

36–18. c *(p. 710)*

36–19. a *(p. 710)*

36–20. a *(p. 711)*

36–21. c *(p. 714)*

36–22. d *(p. 714)*

36–23. d *(p. 715)*

36–24. c *(p. 717)*

36–25. b *(p. 718)*

36–26. c *(p. 719)*

36–27. a *(p. 720)*

CHAPTER 37

37–1. d *(p. 727)*

37–2. b *(p. 727)*

37–3. c *(p. 727)*

37–4. b *(p. 728)*

37–5. d *(p. 728)*

37–6. b *(p. 731)*

37–7. a *(p. 732)*

37–8. d *(p. 733)*

37–9. b *(p. 734)*

37–10. b *(p. 734)*

37–11. b *(p. 734)*

37–12. a *(p. 734)*

37–13. a *(p. 735)*

37–14. a *(p. 736)*

37–15. c *(p. 736)*

37–16. b *(p. 728)*

37–17. d *(p. 732)*

37–18. b *(p. 732)*

37–19. a *(p. 733)*

37–20. d *(p. 734)*

37–21. d *(p. 734)*

37–22. b *(p. 734)*

37–23. d *(p. 734)*

37–24. c (*p. 735*)

37–25. c (*p. 727*)

37–26. b (*p. 727*)

37–27. a (*p. 736*)

CHAPTER 38

38–1. c (*p. 742*)

38–2. c (*p. 744*)

38–3. d (*p. 744*)

38–4. c (*p. 745*)

38–5. d (*p. 745*)

38–6. d (*p. 747*)

38–7. c (*p. 748*)

38–8. a (*p. 749*)

38–9. b (*p. 750*)

38–10. a (*p. 754*)

38–11. d (*p. 754*)

38–12. d (*p. 756*)

38–13. d (*p. 756*)

38–14. a (*p. 751*)

38–15. a (*p. 755*)

38–16. b (*p. 744*)

38–17. c (*p. 749*)

38–18. d (*p. 742*)

38–19. b (*p. 742*)

38–20. c (*p. 743*)

38–21. c (*p. 745*)

38–22. d (*p. 747*)

38–23. b (*p. 749*)

38–24. c (*p. 751*)

38–25. a (*p. 727*)

38–26. d (*p. 754*)

38–27. b (*p. 742*)

INDEX

The numbers following each entry indicate chapter and question numbers. Numbers followed by p refer to the page numbers of the case studies that appear in this book.

INSTRUCTIONS FOR OBTAINING CME

On the following pages are 100 test questions. Please indicate your answers to these questions on the blue answer grid that appears at the end of the book. ANSWERS MUST BE RECORDED IN PENCIL. Complete the CME evaluation form printed on the reverse side. Enclose the completed answer grid and CME evaluation form in the preaddressed envelope along with a check for $20 payable to The University of Texas Southwestern Medical Center in Dallas.

Statement of Educational Need

This study guide was designed to give the reader an understanding of the management of reproductive endocrinology and infertility, which is presented in detail in the *Textbook of Reproductive Medicine, 2nd Edition*. The purpose of this study guide is to assess comprehension and retention of materials covered in the textbook.

In recent years, new data have added substantially to our knowledge of reproductive medicine and have changed many management schemes and practice patterns. This updated information needs to be disseminated to physician in order to help improve recognition and management of reproductive endocrinology and infertility.

Target Audience and Suggested Use of Materials

The said educational materials is comprised of the study guide and case studies for the 2nd Edition of the *Textbook of Reproductive Medicine*. It is suggested that, prior to taking the examination, the participants review the 2nd edition of the *Textbook of Reproductive Medicine*, complete the questions contained in the study guide, and finally complete the test evaluation.

Educational Objectives

After reviewing the above materials, individuals will be able to:
1. Determine their fund of knowledge with regard to basic reproductive endocrinology.
2. Determine the fund of knowledge with regard to clinical reproductive endocrinology.
3. Determine their fund of knowledge with regard to infertility.

CONTINUING MEDICAL EDUCATION QUESTIONS

1. Which of the following best describes the sperm tail consisting of a central axoneme?

    a. 7 + 7 + 2 microtubules
    b. 7 + 7 microtubules
    c. 9 + 9 + 2 microtubules
    d. 11 + 11 + 2 microtubules

2. Capacitation includes which of the following?

    a. binding to the zona pellucida
    b. acrosome reaction
    c. epididymal maturation
    d. all of the above

3. Zona pellucida protein-3 (ZP-3) exhibits which of the following features?

    a. initial binding to sperm
    b. blocks polyspermy
    c. stimulates sperm capacitation
    d. has no known function

4. What is the primary source of progesterone during week 3 of gestation?

    a. cytotrophoblast
    b. granulosa-lutein cells
    c. fetal adrenal
    d. fetal ovary

5. Which of the following hormones decline after the first trimester of pregnancy?

    a. 17β-hydroxyprogesterone
    b. hCG
    c. hPL
    d. all of the above

6. Which of the following are associated with increased human placental lactogen or human chorionic somatomammotropin?

    a. Rh disease
    b. molar pregnancy
    c. diabetes mellitus
    d. all of the above

7. Elevated DHEA-S levels in cord blood are seen in which of the following?

    a. anencephaly
    b. severe pregnancy induced hypertension
    c. congenital syphilis
    d. none of the above

8. Which of the following hormones have been shown to arrest labor in women?

    a. 17α-hydroxyprogesterone
    b. oxytocin antagonist
    c. progesterone
    d. none of the above

9. Endothelin has which of the following effects on uterine smooth muscle?

    a. stimulates contractions
    b. inhibits contractions
    c. no effect
    d. decreases the amplitude of contraction

10. Diakinesis is which stage of prophase of meiosis I?

    a. first
    b. third
    c. fifth
    d. seventh

11. The X chromatin is described by which of the following?

    a. inactive X chromosome
    b. Lyon hypothesis
    c. evaluated by buccal smear
    d. all of the above

12. In autosomal recessive disorders, what is the risk of affected children?

    a. 1:4
    b. 1:3
    c. 1:2
    d. 1:1

13. Which of the following is true in girls with precocious puberty?

    a. constitutional causes are rare
    b. hCG is often elevated
    c. epiphyseal closure is enhanced
    d. breast development prior to age 10

14. Which of the following syndromes are usually associated with amenorrhea?

    a. McCune-Albright
    b. Russell-Silver
    c. Kallmann
    d. Noonan

15. Pseudosexual precocity or peripheral precocious puberty includes which of the following?

    a. hamartomas
    b. hypothyroidism
    c. premature thelarche
    d. all of the above

16. In an individual with true hermaphroditism, which of the following is not associated?

    a. 46,XX
    b. 46,XX/46,XY
    c. 46,XY
    d. 45,X/46,XY

17. An infant is born with sexual ambiguity. The karyotype is 46,XY. Which of the following is correct?

    a. male pseudohermaphroditism
    b. female pseudohermaphroditism
    c. uterus is usually present
    d. none of the above

18. An infant is born with sexual ambiguity. A uterus is not palpated or detected by ultrasound. The karyotype is XY. A stimulation test with hCG is associated with increased testosterone secretion. Which of the following diagnoses is most likely?

    a. 17α-hydroxylase deficiency
    b. 17β-hydroxysteroid dehydrogenase deficiency

    c. testicular regression
    d. 5α-reductase deficiency

19. The coefficient of variation is described by which of the following?

    a. standard deviation ÷ mean
    b. usually less than 10%
    c. precision of the assay
    d. all of the above

20. Monoclonal antibodies include all of the following EXCEPT one?

    a. are more expensive to produce than polyclonal antibodies
    b. are always superior to polyclonal antibodies
    c. involves formation of spleen and myeloma cells
    d. produced by cell lines

21. Which of the following ligands increases cAMP levels?

    a. norepinephrine
    b. hCG
    c. ACTH
    d. all of the above

22. All of the following EXCEPT one are receptors with tyrosine kinase activity?

    a. LH
    b. EGF
    c. PDGF
    d. insulin

23. Which of the following locations is the principle source of GnRH secretion?

    a. ventromedial nucleus
    b. lateral tuberal nucleus
    c. arcuate nucleus
    d. third ventricle

24. Which of the following products of pro-opiomelanocortin (POMC) contains the most amino acids?

    a. ACTH
    b. β-LPH
    c. α-MSH
    d. CLIP

25. All of the following hormones EXCEPT ONE are involved in ductal growth of the breast?

    a. estrogen
    b. progesterone
    c. growth hormone
    d. cortisol

26. Which of the following stimulates PRL secretion?

    a. GABA
    b. TRH
    c. dopamine
    d. testosterone

27. LH secretion is elevated in which of the following stages of life?

    a. fetus during second trimester
    b. infant six months postpartum
    c. menopause
    d. all of the above

28. At which stage of ovarian follicular development does the antral cavity appear?

    a. primary
    b. secondary
    c. tertiary
    d. Graafian

29. In the human ovary which is the preferred pathway for the formation of androgens?

    a. $\Delta 3$
    b. $\Delta 4$
    c. $\Delta 5$
    d. none of the above

30. Which cell type of the ovary exhibits 17α-hydroxylase activity ($P450_{17\alpha}$)

    a. theca
    b. granulosa
    c. stroma
    d. all of the above

31. Which of the following statements is most accurate?

    a. ovulation occurs on day 14
    b. follicular phase — 13 days
    c. luteal phase — 14 days
    d. all of the above

32. Which of the following is primarily observed during the proliferative phase?

    a. stromal edema
    b. gland mitoses
    c. basal vacuolization
    d. pseudodecidual reaction

33. Which of the following are common in Klinefelter syndrome?

    a. increased LH
    b. decreased testosterone
    c. gynecomastia
    d. all of the above

34. Plasma testosterone levels are low in men in which of the following?

    a. marathon runner
    b. marijuana
    c. heroin
    d. all of the above

35. Which of the following are often seen in individuals with Turner syndrome?

    a. hypothyroidism
    b. galactorrhea
    c. eunuchoidism
    d. none of the above

36. Which of the following are associated with estrogen secretion or production in a woman with secondary amenorrhea?

    a. elevated prolactin
    b. ferning pattern of cervical mucus
    c. craniopharyngioma
    d. empty sella syndrome

37. Which of the following is true regarding microadenoma during pregnancy?

    a. 20% of tumors increase in size
    b. PRL levels are good predictors of tumor enlargement
    c. bromocriptine is indicated if enlargement occurs
    d. surgical removal of tumor is often required

38. All the following *EXCEPT ONE* are characteristic of functional hypothalamic amenorrhea?

    a. often overweight
    b. single
    c. intelligent
    d. compulsive behavior

39. A woman presents with acute retro-orbital headache, visual disturbance, and depressed sensorium. Which of the following would explain this group of symptoms?

    a. Sheehan syndrome
    b. isolated gonadotropin deficiency
    c. pituitary apoplexy
    d. all of the above

40. Which of the following thyroid hormones have the greatest contribution to serum triiodothyronines?

    a. T_4
    b. T_3
    c. rT_3
    d. none of the above

41. What is the normal range for TSH?

    a. 0.5–4.5 pg/ml
    b. 0.5–4.5 µg/dl
    c. 0.5–4.5 ng/dl
    d. none of the above

42. In secondary hypothyroidism, which of the following is true?

    a. TSH levels elevated
    b. T_4 levels are low
    c. associated with antithyroid antibodies
    d. all of the above

43. Corticotropin-releasing hormone (CRH) is composed of how many amino acids?

    a. 3
    b. 9
    c. 39
    d. 41

44. Which of the following is true regarding DHEAS?

    a. levels are low following adrenarche
    b. reach a peak at age 50
    c. higher in men than women
    d. none of the above

45. Which of the following is the most frequent cause of Cushing syndrome?

    a. ectopic ACTH
    b. micronodular adrenal hyperplasia
    c. iatrogenic
    d. microadenoma of pituitary

46. In pubertal girls with PCO syndrome, which of the following is true regarding diurnal LH secretion?

    a. no diurnal changes are seen
    b. increases during sleep
    c. increases after awakening
    d. increases after eating

47. All of the following are true regarding women with PCO EXCEPT ONE?

    a. elevated SHBG
    b. increased free estradiol
    c. high LH/FSH ratio
    d. increased androstenedione levels

48. Gonadotropin-releasing hormone agonists have which of the following effects?

    a. lower cortisol levels
    b. lower DHEAS levels
    c. lower androstenedione levels
    d. all of the above

49. Which of the following describes the resting place of hair growth?

    a. catagen
    b. telogen
    c. anagen
    d. nutragen

50. The treatment of choice for hirsutism due to PCOS is which of the following?

    a. GnRH agonists
    b. spironolactone
    c. oral contraceptive
    d. dexamethasone

51. Which of the following isotopes used for radiolabeling has the shortest half life?

    a. iodine[125]
    b. P[32]
    c. tritium
    d. iodine[131]

52. What is the most desirable feature of an antiserum?

    a. high specificity
    b. ability to dilute to low concentration
    c. stability when frozen
    d. low equilibrium constant

53. Which of the following is considered a secretory immune globulin?

    a. IgG
    b. IgM
    c. IgA
    d. IgE

54. Which of the following terms describes the ability of one cell to control another through local mediators within the same gland or organ?

    a. paracrine
    b. juxtacrine
    c. autocrine
    d. endocrine

55. Which of the following hormones is not composed of an alpha and beta chain?

    a. FSH
    b. LH
    c. growth hormone
    d. TSH

56. Somatostatin is a

    a. tripeptide
    b. tetradecapeptide
    c. decapeptide
    d. heptapeptide

57. The gene for which tropic hormone is found on chromosome 6?

    a. ACTH
    b. LH
    c. FSH
    d. prolactin

58. Oxytocin and vasopressin contain how many amino acids?

    a. 3
    b. 10
    c. 8
    d. 13

59. Which of the following hormones stimulates gland development of the breast?

    a. progesterone
    b. estradiol
    c. growth hormone
    d. prolactin

60. Patients with chronic pain syndrome often have drug dependence problems.

    a. true
    b. false

61. Patients with chronic pain syndrome have conditions that are well defined in terms of peripheral nociceptive mechanisms.

    a. true
    b. false

62. In terms of nociceptive biology, once a receptor is activated a state of hyperalgesia is achieved.

    a. true
    b. false

63. Which of the following diseases have been associated with hyperprolactinemia?

    a. histiocytosis X
    b. tuberculosis
    c. syphilis
    d. all of the above

64. Null cell tumors are small endocrine active lesions.

    a. true
    b. false

65. The most common side effect of dopamine agonist therapy is

    a. psychosis
    b. nausea
    c. syncope
    d. cardiac dysrhythmia

66. The hypersecretion of growth hormone is associated with carpal tunnel syndrome.

    a. true
    b. false

67. Patients with eating disorders such as anorexia frequently have elevated levels of reverse T_3.

    a. true
    b. false

68. 15% of body fat is necessary for normal menstrual function.

    a. true
    b. false

69. Among various athletic events, those who swim have the highest rate of ovulatory dysfunction.

    a. true
    b. false

70. The most useful test for determining the state of hypothyroidism is a high sensitivity TSH assay.

    a. true
    b. false

71. The incidence of hypothyroidism is 10%.

    a. true
    b. false

72. The following drugs used to treat symptoms of hyperthyroidism are Propythiouracil and Propranolol.

    a. true
    b. false

73. Patients with polycystic ovary syndrome will have a normal LH/FSH ratio 60% of the time.

    a. true
    b. false

74. Treatment of a normal cycling woman with a GnRH analog starting on day 1 will produce only down-regulation of gonadotropin therapy.

    a. true
    b. false

75. Which of the following is seen in patients with polycystic ovary syndrome?

    a. elevated DHEAS 50% of the time
    b. elevated free testosterone
    c. decreased sex hormone binding globulin
    d. all of the above

76. Women with polycystic ovary syndrome will frequently have an upper limit of normal total testosterone level.

    a. true
    b. false

77. The most common cause of breast discharge is

    a. galactorrhea
    b. infection
    c. ductal papilloma
    d. malignancy

78. Fibroadenomas of the breast are never found as multiple lesions.

    a. true
    b. false

79. The most significant risk factor for breast cancer is which of the following?

    a. a positive family history
    b. smoking
    c. high fat diet
    d. nulliparity

80. Tamoxifen therapy for women with breast cancer has been associated with endometrial hyperplasia, abnormal uterine bleeding, and ovarian cyst formation.

    a. true
    b. false

81. Which of the following states has had mandated coverage for assisted reproductive technology in place for the longest period of time?

    a. Massachusetts
    b. Maryland
    c. Illinois
    d. Texas

82. Conscientious explicit and judicious use of current best evidence in making decisions about the care of individual patients describes cost effective analysis.

    a. true
    b. false

83. Louise Brown was born in Oldham General District Hospital in Lancaster, England, in 1982.

    a. true
    b. false

84. The production of U.S. medical graduates is approximately 17,000 per year.

    a. true
    b. false

85. Ovulation after day 20 is associated with a much lower pregnancy rate than ovulation before day 16.

    a. true
    b. false

86. In women with premature ovarian failure, pre-treatment with GnRH analogs, birth control pills, or Premarin followed by gonadotropin has been consistently successful in inducing ovulation.

    a. true
    b. false

87. Twin gestations are frequently seen during go-nadotropin therapy with estrogen levels 1,000 pg/ml or higher.

    a. true
    b. false

88. In the state of ovarian hyperstimulation, ovaries 10 cm or larger are classified as moderate disease.

    a. true
    b. false

89. Repeat neosalpingostomy of the distal fallopian tube is associated with a 27% pregnancy rate.

    a. true
    b. false

90. The finding of *Mycoplasma hominis* and *Ureaplasma urealyticum* in the uterine cavity or fallopian tube has been associated with a significant decrease in fertility.

    a. true
    b. false

91. Ectopic pregnancy has been associated with which of the following conditions?

    a. fetal exposure to DES
    b. endometriosis
    c. ovulatory dysfunction
    d. all of the above

92. The majority of patients who undergo a trans-cervical tubal cannulization demonstrate tubal patency a year after undergoing the technique.

    a. true
    b. false

93. The most significant factor influencing the success rate in *in vitro* fertilization is maternal age.

    a. true
    b. false

94. A day 3 FSH level of 10 mIU is associated with a decreased pregnancy rate in *in vitro* fertilization cycles.

    a. true
    b. false

95. Women over the age of 35 are likely to abort with fetuses showing a trisomy.

    a. true
    b. false

96. The divorce rate in infertile couples is significantly higher than the population at large.

    a. true
    b. false

97. Adoption has been associated with subsequent conception.

    a. true
    b. false

98. Performance anxiety caused by a postcoital test can be associated with impotence.

    a. true
    b. false

99. 20% of infertility is associated with stress.

    a. true
    b. false

100. The most frequent presentation of Asherman syndrome is amenorrhea.

    a. true
    b. false

Study Guide for Textbook of Reproductive Medicine, 2/E

Marking Instructions

- Use a No. 2 pencil only.
- Do not use ink, ballpoint, or felt tip pens.
- Make solid marks that fill the oval completely.
- Erase cleanly any marks you wish to change.
- Make no stray marks on this form.
- Do not tear or mutilate this form.

● Correct Mark
⊘ ⊗ Incorrect
⊖ ⊙ Marks

1 (A)(B)(C)(D)	26 (A)(B)(C)(D)	51 (A)(B)(C)(D)	76 (A)(B)
2 (A)(B)(C)(D)	27 (A)(B)(C)(D)	52 (A)(B)(C)(D)	77 (A)(B)(C)(D)
3 (A)(B)(C)(D)	28 (A)(B)(C)(D)	53 (A)(B)(C)(D)	78 (A)(B)
4 (A)(B)(C)(D)	29 (A)(B)(C)(D)	54 (A)(B)(C)(D)	79 (A)(B)(C)(D)
5 (A)(B)(C)(D)	30 (A)(B)(C)(D)	55 (A)(B)(C)(D)	80 (A)(B)
6 (A)(B)(C)(D)	31 (A)(B)(C)(D)	56 (A)(B)(C)(D)	81 (A)(B)(C)(D)
7 (A)(B)(C)(D)	32 (A)(B)(C)(D)	57 (A)(B)(C)(D)	82 (A)(B)
8 (A)(B)(C)(D)	33 (A)(B)(C)(D)	58 (A)(B)(C)(D)	83 (A)(B)
9 (A)(B)(C)(D)	34 (A)(B)(C)(D)	59 (A)(B)(C)(D)	84 (A)(B)
10 (A)(B)(C)(D)	35 (A)(B)(C)(D)	60 (A)(B)	85 (A)(B)
11 (A)(B)(C)(D)	36 (A)(B)(C)(D)	61 (A)(B)	86 (A)(B)
12 (A)(B)(C)(D)	37 (A)(B)(C)(D)	62 (A)(B)	87 (A)(B)
13 (A)(B)(C)(D)	38 (A)(B)(C)(D)	63 (A)(B)(C)(D)	88 (A)(B)
14 (A)(B)(C)(D)	39 (A)(B)(C)(D)	64 (A)(B)	89 (A)(B)
15 (A)(B)(C)(D)	40 (A)(B)(C)(D)	65 (A)(B)(C)(D)	90 (A)(B)
16 (A)(B)(C)(D)	41 (A)(B)(C)(D)	66 (A)(B)	91 (A)(B)(C)(D)
17 (A)(B)(C)(D)	42 (A)(B)(C)(D)	67 (A)(B)	92 (A)(B)
18 (A)(B)(C)(D)	43 (A)(B)(C)(D)	68 (A)(B)	93 (A)(B)
19 (A)(B)(C)(D)	44 (A)(B)(C)(D)	69 (A)(B)	94 (A)(B)
20 (A)(B)(C)(D)	45 (A)(B)(C)(D)	70 (A)(B)	95 (A)(B)
21 (A)(B)(C)(D)	46 (A)(B)(C)(D)	71 (A)(B)	96 (A)(B)
22 (A)(B)(C)(D)	47 (A)(B)(C)(D)	72 (A)(B)	97 (A)(B)
23 (A)(B)(C)(D)	48 (A)(B)(C)(D)	73 (A)(B)	98 (A)(B)
24 (A)(B)(C)(D)	49 (A)(B)(C)(D)	74 (A)(B)	99 (A)(B)
25 (A)(B)(C)(D)	50 (A)(B)(C)(D)	75 (A)(B)(C)(D)	100 (A)(B)

CME Evaluation Questionnaire

THE UNIVERSITY OF TEXAS at Dallas
SOUTHWESTERN MEDICAL CENTER

Marking Instructions

- Use a No. 2 pencil only.
- Do not use ink, ballpoint, or felt tip pens.
- Make solid marks that fill the oval completely.
- Erase cleanly any marks you wish to change.
- Make no stray marks on this form.
- Do not tear or mutilate this form.

● **Correct Mark**

⊘ ⊗ **Incorrect**
⊖ ⊙ **Marks**

▶ **SOCIAL SECURITY #**

1. Are you board certified?
○ Yes ○ No

2. What is your specialty?
○ Family Practice
○ Obstetrics/Gynecology
○ Other Medical Specialty
○ Nurse
○ Allied Health Professional
○ Other Health Professional

FOLD HERE ▶

3. How would you classify your type of practice?
○ Private Solo Practice
○ Group Practice
○ Hospital Based
○ Managed Care

4. What is the size of the community or standard metropolitan area where you practice?
○ Rural ○ Under 20,000 ○ 20,001 to 50,000 ○ 50,001 to 100,000 ○ 100,001 to 500,000 ○ Over 500,000

5. How did you learn about this program?
○ Brochure ○ Continuing Ed Internet Home Page ○ Colleague

Please respond as to whether you agree or disagree with the following statements about this continuing education event.

	STRONGLY DISAGREE	DISAGREE	UNDECIDED	AGREE	STRONGLY AGREE
The overall quality of this activity and its educational content were excellent.	○	○	○	○	○
The stated objectives of the activity were met.	○	○	○	○	○
The educational components were clear and well organized.	○	○	○	○	○
Overall the educational components for this activity were excellent.	○	○	○	○	○
The overall material presented in this activity was balanced and unbiased.	○	○	○	○	○

FOLD HERE — FOLD HERE

	STRONGLY DISAGREE	DISAGREE	UNDECIDED	AGREE	STRONGLY AGREE
The content presented was relevant to my practice.	○	○	○	○	○
The activity will have a strong positive impact on the way I practice.	○	○	○	○	○
The content of this activity met my educational needs.	○	○	○	○	○
I would like to learn more about the topic of this activity.	○	○	○	○	○
I would strongly recommend a colleague to attend this activity.	○	○	○	○	○
This activity will have a positive impact on my use of services of the sponsoring institution.	○	○	○	○	○

PLEASE PRINT. If name and address are not legible, CME certificate may not be issued.

NAME AND DEGREE (Please Print)

SIGNATURE

TELEPHONE   FAX

SOCIAL SECURITY NUMBER

ADDRESS   CITY   STATE   ZIP CODE

To apply for CME credit, use the attached, pre-addressed envelope to return this form, both sides completed, with a check for $20.00 to:

Office of Continuing Medical Education • University of Texas, Southwestern Medical Center at Dallas
5323 Harry Hines Blvd. • Dallas, TX 75235-9059